WHAT IS UP DOC? RUMINATIONS OF A SOLO CARDIOLOGIST

Jim,
Thank you so much for agreeing with my brother. It's been great helping to take care of you. Bill 5/1/18

What Is UP Doc?

Ruminations of A Solo Cardiologist

William G. Franklin

No recommendation in this book is meant to be a prescription for any particular individual. One should always check with one's own physician regarding diagnosis, medications, or other treatment recommendations.

Patient names in these stories are fictitious, and remaining potentially identifying details in the cases discussed are obscured to make individuals unidentifiable. Any resemblance to persons living or dead due to such changes is merely a coincidence and unintentional.

Dedication:

This book is dedicated to my mom, who was a boundless source of inspiration

and

To my patients, who honored me with their unending trust

Table of Contents

Dr. Bill

When I met Bill he was a rather typical male college student of the era – cute, funny, athletic, and full of beans. But there was something unique and special about him that I sensed almost right away. (His patients apparently detect and value this). There was something pastoral about him; he exuded a quiet concern for people who are truly in need, and a reassuring almost irreverent confidence that life, while tricky sometimes, is not always as awful as it might seem. Grounded by simple, core beliefs in the value of life and our place in the universe, he felt life should be enjoyed and laughed at wherever possible - even when curve balls have been thrown. In retrospect, it is amazing to me that at age 20, I found that Bill's attitudes towards things were quite similar to those of my grandfather who had been a physician from the turn of the 20th century in New York City and who had regaled me with stories and humor from his own experiences. My Poppa had a sense of confidence that life could be coped with and should be enjoyed. (Life is too important, he'd remind his grandchildren – and no doubt his patients - to be taken too seriously.)

Much like my grandfather, Bill knew he wanted to be a physician from an early age - it was just a feel he had - and he did not deviate from that aspiration even when it seemed that roadblocks were in the way. My grandfather had "enrolled" at Columbia P&S in 1896 to find himself the only student who had not attended college, much less Yale, Princeton or Harvard. 69 years later, Bill who had been an English literature major was told by a chemistry professor at Columbia that he should give up any idea of attending medical school. Yet Bill and Poppa each had set his course as a young man and would see it through against odds that were either real or perceived. And for each, financial profit from a medical career was the last thing on his mind. So, like Poppa, Bill became a physician who grew a large practice that embraced generations and reached across different economic strata. It was as if they paid heed to a calling and were simply doing what they were cut out to do in the first place.

Practicing from 1900 to 1955, Poppa must have encountered any number of changes during his professional life, good and bad. I can recall during a visit to him in a nursing home (he lived until age 99) that he still had his New England Journals by his side and commented to me how doctors of the day knew so much more now, and that he "...couldn't catch their tails running down the street." But he also commented that he had really "known" his patients, and he was less certain from the way cases were being written up in current journals that that was still the ideal (yes, he was reading them at age 99).

Now Bill and several generations of physicians face significant change in the profession and like Poppa, Bill too has an unease that much of the change does not necessarily enhance the profession – does not enhance the practice of medicine – at the same time that more recent terms and phrases (e.g., patient-centered care) suggest that today's doctors are or will be better doctors. It might be hard to distinguish between the inevitable generational divides - processing the passages of time and change that comes with them - from discerning kernels of truth that shouldn't be lost to coming generations.

I pointed out to Bill that given his concerns about the profession – the possible loss of something valuable - it might be a service for him to describe what he thinks goes into being a physician who truly practices "patient centered care." How will people in the future know unless someone attempts to make a record of it? I urged him to write stories that express what he was taught and that he thinks describe the essence of being a good physician even beyond knowledge and competence.

I must have expected something different, more grand, from what he finally sat down to write because the simplicity or absurdity of some of the stories he records here is striking. His tales are episodic, brief, sometimes vivid, and at times, unremarkable. But altogether I think they reveal how human (perhaps "ordinary" is the better word) patients and physicians are – and how intertwined. How "everyday" the reality of illness and healthcare actually is – not the stuff of celebrity and TV! I take from what Bill writes that the physician as clinician is always an *observer* of people - learning from the patients and from every patient encounter. We see that diagnosis can be an art no matter how much book learning a physician has. His stories reveal how much he thinks about what he is working on and trying to fix.

I should not be surprised. Sometimes, Bill might reach over to hold my hand when we are sitting on the couch together and then I'll notice he actually is taking my pulse! Or we are discussing a book or a movie or some current event when he'll pop out with a unique and keen take on a situation that did not occur to me but that on reflection strikes me as "spot on." He watches differently and sees into the essence of things after years of observing people and how they do things in the most stressful or wonderful of circumstances. Learning with the eye, the ear, the heart and mind has produced in him over the years an acute grasp of situation and an ability to sum it up in a way that can be enlightening to whomever might need or want to understand it.

What the medical profession of the future will be like is still of course an unknown and this small collection does not presume as a policy tome even when opinions are bluntly expressed here and there. Bill valued the institutions where he received his medical education and subsequent training, and the teachers whom he believes exhibited outstanding dedication, and humanity, not to mention knowledge. He counts himself as so fortunate to have been allowed to receive his education through and from them.

There will always be change, new knowledge, and improved solutions and treatments in medical care. But if the practice of medicine can continue to include the professionalism and the caring "laying on of hands" that has characterized the best of the profession of the past, then perhaps we shall be lucky in our future. These stories of becoming "Dr. Bill" may provide the reader with some understanding of what that meant.

~J. Franklin

Thank you, Gracie: An Introduction Rewind

I've read and reread my wife's glowing introduction to this opus. I am amazed to hear so many laudatory statements. Could she be hyping the book or perhaps playing me for a new dress, or both? I am like most men: clueless.

It is also of interest that when I was young and available, few females between the ages of 12 and 32 ever showed any interest in me. Now I have a strong following of supporters who are for the most part younger than 12 (my granddaughters) and above 75 years old. Finally, I am appreciated.

One of my favorite jokes is as follows: Suppose I am alone in the forest, standing under an oak tree, and an acorn falls to the ground. If my wife is not present, am I still wrong??? Absolutely everyone answers the question with a resounding, "Yes!!!"

We men are the chosen, clueless servants, lucky and grateful to be included on the ride. Thank you, Jeanne.

Chapter 1: Bill's Introduction: The Golden Days

Even though I was an English major, I have not derived much pleasure from writing itself. My wife, also an English major, insists that I put down on paper some of the amusing and enlightening stories that I have encountered, and some of the lessons I have learned. Medicine has changed dramatically since I entered the University Of Virginia School of Medicine in 1967. Many of the changes have been spectacular whereas others leave something to be desired. Let's see what we might truly value and therefore what we should strive to preserve.

Hindsight

Before leaving home for medical school in Charlottesville, Virginia, I visited Dr. Golden, my ophthalmologist for the 12 years since I was in the fourth grade. I had been told that I was farsighted, and had needed reading glasses since age 9. I needed a new prescription and anticipated an uneventful visit.

Dr. Golden was about 60 years old with gray hair and his own eyeglasses. His office was in the same location on 66th St. in Manhattan, and the furnishings were modest and unchanging. His only employee, his receptionist, was what might have been termed his common-law wife, Mary. This did not change either.

After examining me and writing a new prescription, Dr. Golden walked me to the reception room. There was no separate waiting room with employees walled off or partially hidden by computers. He asked what I was doing this year, and I told him with controlled joy that I was leaving for medical school in a few days. With a very sad look on his face, Dr.

Golden said how sorry he was that I had missed the golden years of medicine. He explained to me how the federal government had passed a Medicare law that would pay for some of the expenses of people over age 65, and he told me that once “they got their foot in the door" the government types would eventually change everything. He was most upset about how doctors would be told how to practice medicine. He wished me good luck and turned and went back into his office and closed the door. His wife - receptionist came around from behind her desk put her arm around me, apologized for “the doctor’s being upset" and reassured me that things would not change that much.

I of course was mystified in spite of being “farsighted;" I had very little notion of politics or government. And I would not have been able to articulate what this kindly couple was demonstrating in regard to a patient-doctor relationship. I had been taking the bus to their office by myself since the fifth grade. My parents knew I would be treated kindly and maturely. The office rarely had more than one person waiting at a time. The doctor was on time and so were the patients. Mutual respect and courtesy, and kindness were the rule of the day and were taught by example, not by a public relations firm.

Chapter 2: The First Day – The First Lesson

On my very first day of medical school in September 1967 in beautiful, then uncongested and peaceful Charlottesville, Virginia, my entire class of approximately 80 students was directed to the auditorium which was to be our classroom for the next two years. I took a seat in the third row and listened closely to welcoming remarks from the Dean, the chief of cardiothoracic surgery, and other eminent university professors. They expounded upon how hard the next two years were going to be and how we had better be attentive to class and our studies if we intended to be around for the third and fourth years - the clinical years. I can't remember most of the names of these prominent individuals or anything substantive that they said.

At the very end of the session they wheeled in an approximately 80-year-old gentleman who was thin and frail, and who spoke relatively softly. He introduced himself simply as Dr. Smith, a recently retired general practitioner who had practiced in Charlottesville for over 50 years. He recalled that when he entered medical school not even insulin was available. A number of chuckles from the audience followed. He then stated that years of reflection had led him to conclude that 90% of what he had learned in medical school was incorrect. There followed at least 30 to 60 seconds of boisterous laughter. When silence was restored, he quickly stated the following: “I don't expect your experience to be significantly different. So study hard, enjoy it, but always keep an open mind." He then turned his old wooden wheelchair and was wheeled away out the door and out of our lives never to be seen by our class again.

I would like to express my heartfelt gratitude to Dr. Smith for taking the time, making the effort, and having the courage, integrity and honesty to clearly state that our taught credos and beliefs are often proven to be dead wrong.

Chapter 3: First Patient; (or, Training Up a Doctor)

As part of a course on physical examination, I was assigned when a second-year medical student in 1969 to a young woman named Trixie Da Leit. I would have guessed that she was 20 years old, looking about 25, whereas I was 23 years old looking 19. I was not allowed to look at her chart so I could not verify anything that she said. I was also instructed to do a complete history and physical exam, and write everything down.

After introducing myself as a medical student I wanted to confirm that she had volunteered or agreed to the interview. She said yes, and gestured to a chair saying, "Make yourself comfortable." There was a Cheshire-cat smile on her face.

I asked her age. She replied "17." I asked her reason for being in the hospital. She replied, "abdominal pain." I asked her where and requested that she point with her finger. With her whole hand she circled her entire abdomen with three concentric circles. I asked if the pain is sharp or dull. She quickly and agreeably responded "yes." I coaxed her to elaborate, and she said sometimes it was sharp and sometimes it was dull. "Had she experienced diarrhea or constipation?" "My goodness, yes," she responded excitedly as though now we were getting somewhere. "Did anything bring on the pain such as eating, changing position, breathing, or having a bowel movement?" "Yes, all of them cause severe pain," she answered enthusiastically. Then her expression became quite serious as she inquired, "Doctor, what do you think is wrong with me?" I told her it was too early to tell yet - knowing full well I would never arrive at a diagnosis. I bit my tongue, and held back from my desire to tell her she was simply full of raspberry preserves. Could she be CIA, I wondered.

I was determined to survive this challenge even if the charade would take two days. It did. She was a master yarn slinger, a student of Mark Twain, and possibly Davy Crockett. She led me on a wild goose chase with 100 twists and turns. She told me her mother was 23 years old, six years her senior, and taught creative writing at the University. I remarked with an even tone that Trixie might do very well following in her mother's footsteps, if she could write. She thanked me and stated she could write wondrously. She said her mother was originally from "Loozeeani" and had walked to Virginia with her six children eight years ago. She was half French and half Cherokee, and made good money on the side palm reading. Trixie volunteered that she had learned a bit from her mother and wondered if I might want my palm read. I thanked her for the offer but declined on the grounds that it was getting late and I had a long, long way to go.

The Review of Systems, a method of inquiry by which one asks 5 to 10 questions regarding each of the systems of the body, was something I dreaded but could not bear to put off overnight. Trixie answered yes to every question. This is called a Positive Review of Systems, a way of designating a patient as being unreliable or unhelpful. At that juncture I had to record three pages of useless questions. For years, I have simply put a "+" for this situation. Most of the time the patient will have only one or two complaints other than the main one - the chief complaint that is the cause for the evaluation.

Medicare however insists that there be a documentation of the review of each of the 10 body systems with a check next to it in order to be reimbursed an inappropriately low amount regardless of the time spent. Never mind that the patient had a Positive Review of Systems, never mind that you have covered more than 10 systems while asking questions during the physical exam. That doesn't count if you didn't check the boxes. Now the hard-working efficient physician has to spend extra time checking boxes or writing unhelpful and distracting notes in order to be reimbursed less each year. But I digress.

For fun and for data that would substantiate the label "Positive Review of Systems," I asked Trixie the following" "Do your teeth ever turn blue? Do you ever see triple? If you hop on your right foot, does your left foot hurt?" She assured me that the answer was yes to all three.

The next day was a breeze. I performed a physical exam in about one hour and found nothing of note. I thanked Trixie profusely, and told her that I could not find anything major of concern but that I was just a student. A real doctor would go over her lab data and review his conclusions with her. She thanked me and said she knew I would be a good doctor because I was a very good listener. As I sprang for the door, she smiled broadly and said "God bless y'all." I was glad one of us had enjoyed the sessions.

Chapter 4: Still NEGATIVE [After All These Years]

Back in the dark ages, in a previous century, in what seems to have been a previous life, I was a humble medical student at the University of Virginia. At the beginning of my third year, armed with the weighty but irrelevant knowledge of the Krebs Cycle and a cursory acquaintance with my toy-like stethoscope, I was released as it were to the wards. I was assigned to three interns and a resident physician. My responsibilities included obtaining a history and performing a physical exam on an average of eight patients every four days. My duties also included drawing approximately six tubes of blood each morning on each of my patients. This took at least one hour and was required before making rounds with the other students, interns, and resident at 7 AM. Hence, I needed to start the day at 6AM.

Some patients had very poor veins which only became smaller and more difficult to "hit" with each day's assault. Frequently, it would take 15 minutes to carefully draw 6 tubes of blood through a very small needle on one patient alone. The lab test results would be returned to the ward by 4 PM. We were expected to have transcribed the numbers in a tabular form on the chart before afternoon rounds began.

After performing these duties for four weeks, it became clear to me that the interns were ordering the same tests for the most part on every patient regardless of the differing illnesses. I inquired quietly of the interns and separately of the resident whether or not all the tests had to be repeated every day, including such tests as the glucose on non-diabetic patients. I also wondered if anyone had noticed that each patient`s blood count had declined so that each of my patients now had the diagnosis of anemia. I was informed that I should not question the orders of the interns as they knew much more about the patients than I did.

Like a dutiful slave, I quietly performed my duties for a few more days. One afternoon however, I had had enough of this mindless bloodletting and decided that I was actually doing harm to my patients. While I was transcribing the data on a 70 year-old debilitated African-American lady, I wrote in the result of her third test in three days for syphilis: "still negative".

The intern showed this to the resident who took me aside to have a heart-to-heart discussion. I reminded him that I had pointed out previously that tests were being ordered mechanically and that this anemic patient was already weak and would soon need a blood transfusion. He agreed finally that there was merit to my observations and promised that the interns and he would listen to suggestions about ordering only those tests that were needed to make day-to-day decisions. He strongly suggested that I refrain from making further comments on the chart as that might provoke a negative response from someone at the top of the totem pole.

I have from that point onward tried to order only those tests that I believe are necessary to make appropriate recommendations regarding patient care. It is clear from my continued contact with medical students and residents that, in spite of the rising costs of health care, there is a continuing tendency to order tests that seem unnecessary and expensive in order to avoid unpleasant criticism, legal, peer-review, or otherwise.

Chapter 5: That's Some Gall Stone

During my second year of medical school in Charlottesville, there was a year-long course in pathology. Part of the course involved hands-on review of "pot cases." We would each be given a large pot with the major organs (of someone who had already died), and we were expected to determine the cause of death.

It was a long day (they all were) and listening to the mundane, monotone presentations of my classmates did not help. My own pot case was exceedingly dull. The heart, lungs, liver, and kidneys were all normal. The only abnormality was a 15 mm diameter gallstone and a tear in the gallbladder. I maneuvered the stone through the rent, into the inferior vena cava, through the right atrium, and right ventricle and out to the left pulmonary artery where it became lodged. When my turn came to present my case, I described the normal organs in a matter-of-fact tone but concluded with the surprise finding of a large calculus (stone) in the pulmonary artery that was the likely cause of death. The pathologist was astounded. He examined the organs and confirmed the other normal findings and remarked how this might be a reportable case. I assured him that it was definitely not reportable because I had taken the liberty of moving the stone to the pulmonary artery in order to stir up some enthusiasm for an otherwise dull, routine case. The patient had likely died of peritonitis and sepsis from the ruptured gallbladder. After my confession, order and solemnity returned to the pot cases.

Since then I have continued to keep an eye out for new findings regarding gallstones, which are 99% cholesterol. Until recently no medicine has seemed to prevent them. Now, however, there are reports that people on statins for lowering cholesterol have a lower incidence of gall bladder surgery. Perhaps a cure is just around the corner.

Chapter 6: Not So Superficial Wounds

When I was in sixth grade, I shared a bathroom with my brother who is four years older than me. He had left a used, uncovered razor-blade on the sink. I was worried that someone might be cut. I thought for a few minutes about my options. I could leave the blade where it was and hope that no one was hurt. I could put it in the medicine cabinet where it could still cause injury. I opted to place it in the bottom of the trash can.

At the time my mother had hired an elderly Russian immigrant, who spoke “broken” English, to help with cleaning: sweeping, vacuuming, washing windows, and, of course emptying the trash baskets. Ana was a dear, sweet, cheerful woman in whose veins flowed the milk of human kindness. I liked her a lot. She was like the interactive, positive grandmother that I never had.

I had no way of knowing but Ana’s method of disposing the trash was not to tilt the basket over the incinerator shoot in our apartment and let gravity do its job but to reach into the basket and grasp whatever was there and thrust it down the shoot. Of course, she grabbed the razor blade and cut the tip of her middle finger. She immediately went to my mother to report the incident. My mother summoned me. Yes, I had put the razor blade in the basket. Ana told me what had happened and showed me her bleeding finger. I was beyond mortified. The last thing I wanted was to cause pain and suffering for anyone, let alone Ana. I apologized, meekly looking down at the floor. I asked what I should have done. My mother said: “It’s simple. Just ask.”

The bleeding stopped with pressure. My mother bandaged the wound. No one ever brought it up again. But I shan't forget. I am still sorry, Ana. My bad. I did not need to take an oath to do no harm. It had already been embedded into my being. Now it was chiseled into my brain.

Thirteen years later, I was in the third year of medical school (19th grade) helping to care for Miss Jane, a comatose lady from a nursing home who at that point remained undiagnosed after a week in the hospital. She had somehow incurred an abscission of her left calf, which had been cleaned with peroxide, treated with antibiotic ointment, and bandaged. I was instructed to change the bandage. Simple enough. Right? Wrong! Whoever had applied the last bandage had wrapped the gauze tightly all around the calf and finished up with knots that brought to mind Alexander the Great's Gordian Knot. Since medical students did not have scissors, I asked the nurse who was assisting me for hers. She produced a pair with sharp tips and I asked her if she could obtain a pair with blunted tips. She indicated that there was not such a pair on this non-surgical ward. I reluctantly proceeded to slowly and gently raise the edge of the bandage and slide the lower blade of the scissors an inch or so forward and cut the bandage. I lifted the bandage further and was able to see that I had cut the poor lady's skin resulting in a half-inch shallow incision. I was devastated. I told myself aloud that it was inexcusable. The nurse tried the blame the scissors and soften my grief by telling me the cut was minor and would heal. She might also have said that the lady was likely to die. Regardless, I told her that it was terrible. I sent her off to find appropriate scissors and a suturing kit. I removed the bandage and used one stitch to close the wound. I instructed the nurse to use the peroxide and antibacterial cream and wrap the area loosely and tape the end of the gauze, not tie it. I then wrote a progress note on the chart describing the inadvertent mishap and the subsequent stitching. I informed my resident supervisor and showed him the note. He asked: "Lesson learned?" I said: "Yes, never do anything, no matter how simple it may appear, without obtaining the proper equipment." I told him how devastated I was. He looked up from his chair and replied: "I'm positive you will see much worse at some point in your career." That was not cheering. There was no penance either. I was reminded of Ana and felt even worse. I knew my parents would have been disappointed, but not as disappointed as I was.

Years later, there was a poster in the medical records department at (then) Arlington Hospital that reminded me of these errors. It showed Charlie Chaplin sitting in an old automobile tire, floating down a river, wearing a Top Hat and a tuxedo, smoking a cigar, reading the NY Times, with his legs crossed. The caption underneath this scene read something like this:

Good judgement comes from wisdom.

Wisdom comes from knowledge.

Knowledge comes from experience.

Experience comes from bad judgement.

Bad judgement comes from lack of wisdom.

Chapter 7: In the Nick of Time

During my third year of medical school, one of my rotations was in Obstetrics and Gynecology. I was assigned one day to participate in the case of a pregnant woman who was in the early stage of labor. Her contractions were at first regular but weak. I was supposed to provide her with ice chips or a wet cloth for her dry mouth and empathy and encouragement for her discomfort. A fetal monitor was in place and I was to stay in the room and notify the nurse and resident physician if the heart rate decreased alarmingly at any time. I was told I could lie down in the second bed in the room, that the alarm would go off if there was a problem. Hours went by with some progress but the lady was not fully dilated at midnight. It was not easy to doze off because the Muzac kept playing a song from a Tom Jones Album (What's New Pussycat?) over and over again. I was reminded of my college fraternity initiation during which there was a continuous playing of Bolero, for hours on end.

Suddenly, at about 3 AM, the fetal monitor alarm went off loud and clear. The baby's heart rate had gone down to 100 and was not bouncing back up. I called for the nurse who came immediately. She then ran and wakened the chief resident who came immediately and then assembled the team of nurses. The patient was informed that the baby was in danger and we had to act immediately. The heart rate was still too low. It took a few minutes to wheel her into the operating room and transfer her to the table. I was told to start getting necessary materials out of the cabinets and dump them quickly on the nurse's stand. I know anesthesia was there but I can't say that they administered any anesthetic. The chief resident was gowned and gloved and asked the nurse to note the time: 3:05 AM. He then made a long midline incision and sliced open the uterus and extracted the baby. Very shortly, the baby cried. The nurse noted the time: 3:08 AM. The obstetrics resident said cooly: "Incision to baby crying. That's pretty good. Thanks everyone." He went about stitching things up, which took considerable more time than 3 minutes. Afterwards the mom was able to hold what appeared to be a nice pink, alert baby with an Apgar score of 9 at 1 minute.

I have seen some dramatic events over the years but nothing outranks this emergency C-section. The danger was real. There was no time to debate. The only appropriate decision was made. Surgery was performed rapidly and with great skill and much concern. Statistics have little place in this situation. No one has a crystal ball, but without an immediate operation the child may have incurred brain damage. It would seem to me that it would be wiser and safer to deliver in a hospital situation rather than at home. Why take chances?

Chapter 8: Diarrhea (A Red Herring)

I volunteered as a student in June and July of 1972 to work in Fort Defiance, Arizona on the Navajo reservation and then returned to the reservation voluntarily in 1973 until 1975 as a physician. The military draft had been eliminated by President Nixon. I was stationed at the United States Public Health Service Hospital in Shiprock, New Mexico located in the four corners region where New Mexico, Arizona Utah, and Colorado come together. The area is recognizable in many commercials by the volcanic rock formation that appears similar to the rock of Gibraltar and is known by the Navajo people as Tsé bit' a' í.

There were 20 doctors at the hospital, and so we were on call at the hospital all night long about every three weeks. People would drive as much as two hours to Shiprock over sometimes muddy, rough dirt roads across 100 miles of barren land to get to the healthcare promised to them 150 years ago and guaranteed by the sacred treaty signed by the tribe and the United States.

One night, I had finished seeing the usual deluge of visitors to the emergency room, and had gone to sleep around midnight. I was awakened at 2 AM by the nurse who told me that a father was in the emergency room with his 12-year-old son who had been having diarrhea for 2 to 3 days. They had driven 2 1/2 hours and covered 120 miles. Possible diagnoses included food poisoning - perhaps salmonella or shigella. These are common on the reservation where traditional Navajo dwellings called hogans, composed of wood and dirt, did not usually have electricity or refrigeration. (No two-car garages to boast about.)

Neither the father nor the son spoke English. The nurse interpreter explained that the boy had produced 10 loose stools that day and 20 to 30 over the previous day. He had not had any fever or abdominal pain or vomiting. I went over this repeatedly because the history is supposed to be the most important element of the initial encounter.

The boy was lying still on the examining table only speaking when addressed and answering with short phrases in Navajo. I listened to his lungs, heart, and abdomen and noted hyperactive bowel signs consistent with diarrhea. I bent his legs at the knees, and told him through the nurse to try to relax as I started to examine his abdomen with light palpation in the upper abdomen. I gradually worked my way down to the right lower quadrant (RLQ). I watched his face as I examined him and there was a slight wince and squinting of the eyes when I pressed on the RLQ. The spot is called McBurney's Point and it marks the most common site of pain from an inflamed appendix. But that didn't make sense; the boy insisted that he had diarrhea, no fever or chills, and no pain in the abdomen unless I pressed on the RLQ. I re-examined his abdomen going from place to place in differing patterns. He had tenderness when letting up, called rebound tenderness, throughout the abdomen. Nothing fit the medical school lectures, the textbooks, or Copley's famous The Acute Abdomen.

It would have been easy to admit the lad, start intravenous antibiotics, and ask for surgical consultation in the morning but the potentially life-threatening presence of a rupturing appendix still disturbed me.

I called the surgeon and apologized for waking him. He was Dr. Taylor McKenzie, the first Navajo physician (as opposed to a Navajo Medicine Man), and fortunately he lived only a few houses away. I explained about the diarrhea, the lack of fever, the normal white blood count (white blood cells fight infection and the count should be high if appendicitis is present). I told him I examined the abdomen multiple times and that the boy was consistently tender over the RLQ. I asked Dr. Mackenzie to evaluate him and consider emergency surgery. He arrived shortly and took the patient into surgery. I went back to sleep.

The next morning Dr. McKenzie was strolling down the hallway with a cup of coffee in hand and the usual straight-faced and calm speech characteristic of his people. I had still thought the most likely explanation was food poisoning but that I couldn't chance that for the patient's sake.

Dr. McKenzie calmly told me that it was appendicitis and that as soon as he had isolated and contained it, it BURST! I asked him for some explanation of the diarrhea, and he had none. He told me never to be hesitant to wake him or any other physician in the future. I wanted to call up to heaven to thank Dr. Smith from Charlottesville for his sage advice. If I had not questioned the validity of what I had been taught, a young man could have died. I don't remember the boy's name but I want to think the last name was Chee. (That is common on the reservation; the first name often changes when a boy reaches maturity.) I like to remember the boy of few words as Hosteen - Navajo for “man.” Hosteen Chee would be 49 years old today. I like to think when someone has been snatched from death's door and given a new lease on life that it is appropriate to say in a very subtle Native American Way, “Have a great day, Hasteen Chee, Ya’ateeh. It is well.”

Chapter 9: Aunt Minnie

One afternoon on the Navajo reservation, I returned home one block from the hospital in Shiprock, New Mexico for lunch. I walked up to the door, and the babysitter walked quickly down the steps past me to her mother, aunt, and sister who were waiting in the car. Marina Tsosie, part Navajo and part Ute, was 18 years old and was so laconic she made the entire state of Maine look chatty. I asked her if everything was fine and she replied yes, and got in the car and left.

I entered the living room area to find my overactive, always- in- motion, one-year-old daughter sitting perfectly still on the couch with a book. At first I was pleasantly surprised. I sat down right next to her and leaned over to give her a kiss. Usually she would throw her arms around my neck, choke me half to death, and then climb on my back for a piggyback ride up and down the block. Today she moved away slightly. I put my lips to her forehead, a way of assessing her temperature – a technique my mother, a nurse, had taught me years before (I was amazed as a teenager to discover how few young ladies realize the value of this). Nowadays if you use this technique you would be labeled an outlier or pervert and at best put on probation). But I digress, again.

My daughter's right thigh looked red, felt warm and was definitely sensitive to the touch. She would not stand and walk on it. I immediately carried her up to the emergency room. The doctor on duty had gone to lunch so I asked the nurse Daisy Descheenie to get Lisa's chart. I started to check Lisa's ears, throat, lungs, heart, and abdomen to be complete. I was wondering if blood tests should be the next step or should I go straight to an x-ray of the leg when Daisy re-entered laughing. I had never seen a Navajo woman laugh this loud, trying to cover her mouth to modulate her hoots. She laid Lisa's chart on the counter and pointed to an entry three hours earlier documenting the administration of Lisa's routine DPT vaccine.

My reputation as a diagnostician spread rapidly throughout the hospital. I was just a little pleased at my new-found fame. Many people who had never commented when passing me in the hallway before now smiled broadly directly at me, which was uncharacteristic of Navajo at that time, and joyfully said "Good morning, Dr. Franklin!" When I later told my wife of the day's happenings, she too was amazed and amused.

I was at that time teaching Navajo high school graduates what they needed to know to be community health medics. Their function would be a cross between that of a visiting nurse, a primary care doctor making a house call (a what?), and a rescue squad medic. I had set up a schedule of afternoon lectures and required reading with participation of all the doctors – surgeons, pediatricians, internists, and obstetrician-gynecologists. After graduation, each community health medic would be assigned to a 50 to 75-mile area. They were to meet, check out, and familiarize themselves with as many people in the outlying communities as possible. I taught them to be observant and to get to know their patients. They needed to be responsible, and follow up regularly. All of this was a part of "continuity of care." Just as I had noted something different about my daughter, they would be able to notice something that no one else could know if they were seeing the patient for the first time or not interacting regularly.

This had been explained to me years before during the physical diagnosis course in my second year of medical school in Charlottesville in the following way: someone may ask you who a person was who just turned the corner and was out of view; after a second's glimpse, you may be able to reply immediately and confidently, "That was my Aunt Minnie." You may not be able to describe her in words but you know your Aunt Minnie when you see her. You don't need a randomized double-blind study.

There have been numerous times when I have noted a significant difference in the patient that others had not appreciated. One time I noted slightly bulging eyes in a colleague who had just entered an auditorium and sat down across the room from me. I relayed through another colleague a recommendation that he have his thyroid tested. He was tested and found to be hyperactive with Graves' disease. Neither the patient nor his family had had a clue that he was ill.

Today, continuity of care is on the endangered species list and soon may be extinct. Primary care doctors are not paid enough nor do they have as much energy after seeing 20 to 40 patients a day in the office. Consequently, they are yielding to the practice of hospitals hiring hospitalists, doctors employed by the hospital, who take charge in place of the primary care doctor when the primary care doctor's patient is admitted to the hospital. These physicians have no office, have never seen the patient before, and likely will never see the patient again unless the patient is readmitted.

Hospitals are convinced that hospitalists discharge patients sooner than the average primary care doctor does and Length of Stay (LOS) data is required reportable data. The impact of the DRG system instituted under President Reagan has been the loss of over 500 hospitals nationwide since 1983. (With the DRG (a diagnostic related group), a hospital is reimbursed the same amount, for example for pneumonia regardless of whether the patient stays in the hospital one day or 30 days). The disappearance of independent non-profit hospitals has steadily continued.

Survival and cutting costs are the bottom line, and continuity of care is no longer discussed. How the newer "patient-centered care" is supposed to be a suitable remedy for the loss is unclear to me. But Aunt Minnie will not have one single primary care Doctor; she will encounter many healthcare providers. Only a very small percentage of medical school graduates are even contemplating primary care, and more and more are choosing practice avenues which will include reduced schedules, restricted call, and sharing of patients. The idea that a single primary care doctor will be responsible for one's care is almost at an end and doctors will no longer recognize Aunt Minnie nor realize something is amiss even when she is sitting in their office right in front of them.

Chapter 10: Friday Afternoon

Friday afternoon is different from other afternoons. There always seems to be someone who calls up with symptoms that are days old or require complex arrangements. Fridays simply cannot be trusted. So it was one Friday afternoon when I was quietly walking through the Emergency Ward (EW) entrance to see my patients upstairs that an EW doctor asked me for a “quick consultation" on a patient.

It was simple enough, he explained: a 55-year-old man had experienced sharp chest pain under the breast bone lasting from 6 AM to 11 AM - too long for angina, reversible heart ischemia (reduced blood flow) and long enough for heart attack to be apparent. However, the ECG (electrocardiogram) was entirely normal and the cartilages of his chest were tender to touch, the implication being that the patient had inflammation of the cartilages and ribs, a benign condition called Costochondritis. I interviewed and examined the patient, and indeed felt the sharp pain and tender chest wall were due to Costochondritis and not a heart attack. However, there was one problem. A blood test had been ordered and it was abnormal, barely. The test was a muscle test called the CPK and the result was 35 with a normal of 33 at that time. It certainly could have come from chest wall muscle but it could also have been from his heart. The patient at that point wanted to go home and regretted that he had even come to the EW. The EW doctor had expected me to agree that the patient could go home. The character of the pain, sharp as opposed to dull, and the presence of chest wall tenderness were taught to be non-cardiac and that had been my experience up to that point. However, the abnormal blood test caused me to be wary, and to decide that caution dictated that the patient stay overnight.

The next day the EKG showed a large heart attack, and blood tests now confirmed this to be true. The patient underwent coronary angiography demonstrating multi-vessel coronary artery disease (atherosclerosis), and subsequently was referred for coronary artery bypass surgery. The patient could easily have been discharged home and died. Then a lawyer could have asked one question: "Is a CPK of 35 normal, Doctor?"

Thank you once again, Dr. Smith!

Chapter 11: Stomach Ulcers and Stomach Cancer: I'm not drinking that! Are you crazy?

For hundreds of years, doctors have struggled to determine the causes of stomach ulcers and stomach cancer. At times the causes have been attributed to personality, stress, diet, and even blood type. There was evidence that people with blood type O were more prone to stomach ulcers whereas type A was associated with stomach cancer. This was an association that was included in questions on medical board exams and licensing tests.

Approximately 25 years ago, an Australian gastroenterology fellow wondered if a germ might be the culprit. He inquired of pathologists if they had seen germs or cultured germs from stomach specimens. He was told that germs were sometimes seen but they had never been cultured.

So on his own, Dr. Barry Marshall started to plate out specimens on a multitude of tissue cultures. For months, he turned up nothing. Then one night he was interrupted before he could put his specimens in an incubator. He left the laboratory only to return in the morning to the amazing discovery that a germ had grown. It was a new germ that had been hiding in people's stomachs for centuries. He called the germ HELICOBACTER PYLORI (H. PYLORI for short).

Nobody believed him. He was often rejected when applying to present his data at international conferences. Finally, after 10 years of rejections, he drank a concoction of H. pylori, infected himself, underwent an endoscopy, and treated and cured himself. The world stopped and listened.

It is now established that a majority of stomach ulcers are attributable to H. pylori and that over 95% of stomach cancers are a result of this germ. There is a less frequent kind of stomach cancer called MALT which can sometimes be cured with an antibiotic, tetracycline.

H. pylori lives in the soil. It is present according to Dr. Marshall in 80% of Russians and 20% of Americans. An American couple who adopt a Russian child typically becomes positive within six months.

H. pylori can now be screened for with a stool test, a breath test, and a blood test. A gastroenterologist may perform an endoscopic procedure to look down into the stomach and obtain specimens for culture and microscopic evaluation.

Occasionally, I hear about a case of stomach cancer or ulcers at a conference, at lunch with colleagues, or from the patient. I am surprised that no one has recounted this story, and advised family members to undergo screening. The numbers of people with stomach cancer or ulcers could be significantly reduced.

This is truly a remarkable story, an incredible breakthrough. Dr. Marshall deserves the Nobel Prize. We should take note that Dr. Marshall did not accept the common beliefs about ulcers. We should be amused that the discovery depended on chance (serendipity). The open mind is more likely to accept chance discoveries. His work was not funded by a government or a major research Institute. It depended for the most part on Dr. Marshall's intuition, persistence, and the courage not only to stand up at conferences and be laughed at but also the courage to risk his own health in order to convince others. I would simply add: “Well done, and thank you."

Chapter 12: My Mother's Bowels

There was a time when I used to receive some rather unusual calls after hours. One night a Mr. Flush called, at about 2 AM, and explained that he was "... having trouble with his mother's bowels." The man went on to explain that his mother had been having diarrhea for two days without any pain or other symptoms. I had not turned on the light so my wife could not see that I had covered the receiver with my hand before pretending to reply to the gentleman "It is my firm policy never to mess with *my* mother's bowels and you should find something better to do at 2 AM." What I actually said to the caller when I uncovered the receiver to speak to the gentleman was to suggest that Kaopectate might be helpful, and I offered to call a pharmacy. He replied that there were no pharmacies open at that hour where he lived and he wasn't about to drive 10 miles. I asked him why he had called me if not for some medicine. He answered that he thought I might know of some home remedy. I asked him if he had any champagne available. Surprised, he responded excitedly that he did but he didn't know champagne helped diarrhea. I advised him that the champagne was for him and that the cork was for his mother. By the time, he finished the bottle of champagne, perhaps a drugstore would be open but he would best have someone else drive him there.

Chapter 13: Ass – Frontwards or Sitting on Your Money Literally Can Be a Pain in The Butt

A phrase we would all like to use more frequently is "Get off your butt." Occasionally this can be very important healthwise.

Many men for unknown reasons place their wallet (which astoundingly is always far bigger than my wallet or than wallets used to be in 1960) in their back pockets and sit for hours each day. This causes undue pressure on the sciatic nerve with subsequent shooting pain down the leg or numbness sometimes all the way to the foot. Often these unfortunate souls are extensively evaluated and undergo x-rays of the back, the hip, or the knee, or even nerve conduction studies which are not fun. Every six months or so I have the pleasure of telling someone, "Get off your butt" or better yet: "Now, give me your wallet." In less than a month after removing the culprit from the rear pocket and moving it to the front or side pocket, symptoms resolve and the patient can then walk normally.

Recommendations:

1. I suggest that Congress pass a law banning back pockets in men's pants. This would improve health in general, reduce healthcare costs, and also reduce pickpocketing. Congress will be remembered as the one Congress that actually did something.

2. The pocket makers of the world or the growers of cotton and producers of wool might object. There will have to be some form of monetary compensation for them or else the whole bill would fall victim to a threatened filibuster.

Chapter 14: Losses, Ann Arbor

Almost every physician experiences losses, patients dying in spite of one's best efforts. These can be very painful depending on the circumstances.

Early in my medical training, a lady came all the way from South America for evaluation of her heart condition. Her name was Señora. She was a young adult, not unattractive, and exceedingly gentle. She had incurred acute rheumatic fever following a strep throat at age 12. She had been short of breath since then and could not walk 30 yards on level ground.

Señora was accompanied by her husband who was an American citizen employed by the government. He was soft-spoken, courteous, kind, and gentlemanly. He was devoted to his wife. She was unable to have children and she was his only living relative. The evaluation and treatment took place over a 2 to 3 week hospitalization with chest x-rays, ECGs, cardiac catheterization, digitalis and diuretics. After optimizing care, the decision was made to proceed with open heart surgery and mitral valve replacement. I had rounded on Señora twice a day, with her husband acting as interpreter. She identified with me for some reason and so did her husband, perhaps because I had played soccer in high school and college and was able to discuss her country's World Cup championships with them. On the morning of surgery I came by her room at 7 AM but was unable to speak to her because she was otherwise occupied. I had a number of other patients to see. When I doubled back to her room she had already left for the operating room. The next thing I heard at noon was that the operation had ended disastrously because her heart tissue was stretched so thin and was so frail that suture tore through it. She could not be saved. She was pronounced dead on the table.

I looked all around for her husband but he had left the hospital. When I arrived at home at 7 PM my wife seeing my great distress suggested I look in the telephone book and call all the local m/hotels until I found her husband. I did that, found him, and spoke to him for almost an hour. He was devastated. Always the gentleman however, even through his tears, he thanked me and the hospital for their efforts. He said his wife had a premonition that she would never return to her country and so he was not surprised. He was going to head for his home the next morning. I hope our talking gave him some comfort. I have never forgotten how they faced death with grace, dignity, and love. I have never forgotten how that death of a patient felt.

Chapter 15: Coffee, Mate?

One night in 1971 during my internship at the University of Michigan, I was stationed at Detroit Metropolitan Hospital. It was 3 A.M. I was sitting at the nurses' station in the ICU writing an admission note on a 60 year-old lady with a gastrointestinal bleed, probably an ulcer of the stomach, probably caused by aspirin (the leading cause of hospitalization due to a medicine [ibuprofen ranks number 2]).

As I was concentrating on my note, a co-intern from Australia came around the corner half-asleep, totally disheveled, yawning widely, querying: "Where is the coffee, Bill?" I did not look up or stop writing. I simply responded in a normal voice: "Dunno." To this he repeated: "Come on, Bill, tell me where the coffee is." I replied calmly: "I really don't know." Russell (Why not?), now almost totally awake, raised his voice and crowed. (He crowed. He did.) "You better tell me where the coffee is. You are beginning to piss me off." I patiently informed him that I didn't know since I didn't drink coffee. "In fact, I can't stand the taste of coffee." His eyes were wide open by then as he pronounced: "I can't believe it. How can you be wide awake at 3 A.M. without coffee?" I told him that there was this 60-year-old lady who was trying to bleed to death, and I was not about to let that happen on my shift (33 hours). I pointed out that he looked wide-awake right then and probably didn't need coffee and that the coffee would likely interfere with his ability to get back to sleep.

Since then I have seen on television or been told that most people cannot tell the difference between decaf and regular coffee. There is probably a booming coffee business based on the placebo effect. Caffeine generally raises the heart rate and the blood pressure and provokes palpitations. Many patients have their palpitations resolved after eliminating caffeine from their coffee or sodas.

Chapter 16: Identity Theft – HIPAA Take Note

One day in the office, a day like any other day, the nurse opened the door to the waiting room and called out "Mrs. HIPAA." There were a few middle-aged ladies present, but one raised her hand immediately, jumped up, and proceeded to the examining room. The nurse obtained baseline data including the weight and blood pressure, chatting with her and asking questions such as, "How have you been feeling, Mrs. HIPAA?" She responded, "Very well, thank you." The nurse left the room and I entered asking "How are you feeling, Mrs. HIPAA?" She answered "Very well indeed. But I was expecting to see Dr. Blank." I looked at her chart and noted that she had been one of my patients but had not been back for many years. I said "Certainly, whatever you wish." I left the room, gave the chart to the nurse, and went into another room to see someone else.

When I came back out in the hallway the nurse said "It's okay. Mrs HIPAA will see you now." Confused, I reentered the room with the chart again, only to find a different lady – one whom I easily recognized. Upon completion of the visit, I left the room and asked the nurse how the first patient, the wrong patient, ended up in my examining room with the other lady's chart.

The nurse recounted what the first patient said when the nurse had asked her why she said yes, she was Mrs. HIPAA. Well, the lady told my nurse, "I was tired of waiting for Dr. Blank, and I liked the other patient's name." The nurse also asked the real Mrs. HIPAA if she had heard her name called earlier and seen the other lady respond to it. She replied "Yes, but this other lady said she was me so I just sat down and waited."

I am sure that the electronic medical record will eliminate these kinds of errors, particularly when it's a full moon.

Chapter 17: House Call

In 1980 I admitted a patient with congestive heart failure (CHF) who was brought from his home by the rescue squad without his glasses. His shortness of breath improved considerably overnight so that by the next day he was much inconvenienced and could not even see the television let alone the newspaper. I inquired of the nursing staff and the social workers if there was someone or some mechanism to retrieve the gentleman's eyeglasses. The answer was, “No." I went back into the patient's room and asked if he had relatives or friends who could go to his house and find the glasses. The answer was again “No.” I then asked if he would like me to go to his house and bring him his glasses. The answer was a surprised but delighted “Yes.” He gave me his keys and directions to his house, and told me where to look for the glasses. Late in the day I brought him his glasses and he was most appreciative.

Now a house call as portrayed in recent years on television by Dr. House would involve a break-in and a search for abused substances or toxins. Goodbye to trust and peace of mind.

For the first three years of private practice in Arlington I made house calls for patients who were essentially homebound. I was amazed to learn that Medicare reimbursed me a nominal amount whereas they would remunerate nurses quite a bit more for a visit. Nonetheless, I continued to make occasional visits. It was not about the money. However, since there was no portable EKG machine, I was possibly opening myself up to criticism if the patient later had a heart attack. I would have been asked why I had not sent the patient to the ER. So much for house calls!

Chapter 18: Buying a Picture at Face Value

Sometime late in 1983, I was leaving Fairfax Hospital after seeing a few patients there. I was on the elevator heading down when a lady with an oversized box got on, looking forlorn, on the verge of tears. I asked her what the problem was. She said that she had a number of pictures that she had tried to sell to the Hospital but they had declined.

I knew I was moving my office on January 1, 1984, to its present location next to the hospital in Arlington. I figured I would need at least three pictures for each of four examining rooms.

I asked the lady to show me her pictures. They were photographs of landscapes, covered bridges, mountains, seascapes, old mills, and panthers. They had been "enhanced" to bring out minute details such as droplets on waves in the ocean. Each was mounted in a plain, brown frame. They were great.

She told me they were $25 each. I told her I had no money with me but she could come to my office. I would buy 12 of them. She was delighted. Her sad expression quickly transformed into a big, broad grin from ear to ear.

I was pleased to have helped at least one person that day.

I still have a number of her pictures in the examining rooms. Patients frequently comment on their beauty.

Chapter 19: Heart Attacks: Then and Now

In the 1950s, a medicine called INH was created, tried out on first on the Navajo reservation, and then released to the general population. The results were nothing short of miraculous. Within 10 years, tuberculosis (TB) was no longer the number one killer, a distinction it had held for centuries. TB sanatoria gradually became unnecessary and were closed one by one. The last one in Virginia, Blue Ridge Sanatorium in Charlottesville, closed within a year or two of my rotation there as a fourth-year medical student in 1971.

The new and presently number one killer became atherosclerosis (cholesterol blockages of large arteries). An alternative name is arteriosclerosis (blockages of small arteries called arterioles). Many simply use the lay terminology "hardening of the arteries." The number one consequence of this disease is heart attacks, known as "coronaries" in the 1950s. "Coronaries" was actually short for coronary thrombosis which meant a blood clot within a cholesterol- narrowed artery.

In 1969 when I first started helping to take care of patients, there was felt to be no medication to prevent or treat heart attack victims. Sublingual (under the tongue) nitroglycerin was available but felt to be too dangerous because it would lower the blood pressure. Intravenous heparin was available but thought to be inappropriate since it did not dissolve clots already present. In fact, the only treatment was absolute bed-rest, which when carried out for several weeks would result in approximately 20% of patients acquiring shoulder-hand syndrome, with pain, numbness, and lack of strength usually in the left arm. This would mysteriously resolve with activity and be totally preventable if bed-rest was limited to three weeks. Cautiously physicians gradually reduced the period of rest to three days by 1976.

In 1976, I began my two-year cardiology fellowship at Georgetown University Hospital, and learned from world-renowned pathologists that a “coronary" was not really a “coronary thrombosis" because there was no clot demonstrated on post-mortem exam. We were taught that at least 25% of heart attacks resulted in clots inside the left ventricle (pumping chamber) which would then travel to the brain, the spleen, the kidneys, virtually anywhere. At least an additional 5% of patients would develop phlebitis (clots in the veins of the legs) and pulmonary emboli (clots in the lungs). Bed rest was the likely culprit in causing clots in the legs which would then travel to the lungs.

In 1978, I began private practice in cardiology in Arlington, Virginia. I joined Dr. Raymond Hoare, a super smart, astute, caring product 10 years earlier of the same Georgetown cardiology division run by the revered Dr. Proctor Harvey.

One of my first patients was a middle aged gentleman admitted with a heart attack that was considered small since his ECG did not have Q waves (large downward deflection shaped like a V) or ST elevation (flat upright horizontal table-like forms). There were T wave inversions inferiorly (downward hole-like; on the under surface of the left ventricle). The CPK blood test was about 60 - not quite twice normal. This everyone thought, myself included, was a small heart attack that would have minimal residual effect. Shockingly, a few hours later, the man lost the pulse in his right arm. I began IV heparin (an anticlotting medicine) immediately. Because there was no cardiac catheterization laboratory at Arlington Hospital at that time, the patient was transferred to Fairfax Hospital for angiography. The test demonstrated a clot in his right arm above the elbow which later dissolved. More importantly, it demonstrated a blockage of the right coronary artery that was 98% of the way across the blood vessel. A picture of the pumping chamber was normal, confirming that the heart attack was a small one. There was no visible clot in the pumping chamber. Since angioplasty (balloon dilatation) was not available in this country until 1981, the patient underwent coronary artery bypass surgery (CABG) and a major heart attack was averted.

From that time on, I prescribed heparin to almost all my heart attack patients in order to prevent not only emboli, strokes, phlebitis, and pulmonary emboli, but also to maintain patency of the coronary artery, which had to have been at risk of clotting off. This latter conclusion flew in the face of previous teaching.

Fortunately, in 1980 a courageous group of cardiologists and surgeons in Spokane, Washington, decided to break with present recommendations and perform angiograms on heart attack patients immediately upon arrival. They discovered that the culprit arteries had clotted off and that immediate CABG could save lives. Hallelujah!

Before 1970 there were 1.6 million heart attacks in the USA with a 50% mortality rate after reaching the hospital. The predominant cause of death was an abnormal heart rhythm, usually ventricular fibrillation (VF), a totally irregular and inefficient beating of the pumping chamber. In the 1960s, doctors in Belfast Northern Ireland, decided to rush to the scene of a heart attack victim, inject in the thigh a medicine, lidocaine, to prevent or treat the abnormal rhythm, institute CPR (cardiopulmonary resuscitation) and admit the patient to monitored ICU rooms where IV lidocaine, and defibrillation would be more quickly administered. The institution of coronary care units resulted in a decrease in mortality from 50% to approximately 25% post hospital arrival. UVA hospital was among the first to initiate a mobile CCU (a precursor of today's rescue squad) under the guidance of an aggressive, energetic cardiologist named Dr. Richard Crampton,* whom we fondly referred to as Dr. Dracula for his long (below the knees) white coat and hair halfway down the neck (long for those days). Arlington Hospital was the fourth in the country to open a CCU.

During my residency at the University of Michigan Hospital in 1975, I reviewed the charts on heart attack patients for the previous five years. Shockingly, the data indicated that the average time from onset of symptoms to entering the EW was 24 hours. Since then, this interval has gradually declined to approximately 2 hours on average. This is a tremendous improvement but still leaves much to be desired. The longer heart muscle is deprived of normal blood flow, the more damage is done and the greater the risk of death.

Angioplasty of the coronary arteries (PTCA) was introduced in the 1970s in Switzerland by Dr. Andreas Gruentzig. Dr. Gruentzig later moved to Atlanta and ran instructional courses on PTCA at Emory University. Since then, emergency PTCA for heart attacks spread nationwide, and has saved hundreds of thousands of lives. This has been an incredible and exciting odyssey.

In a matter of 30 years, we have gone from nothing but supportive care for heart attack patients to coronary angioplasties and multiple life-saving medications. It is nothing short of a miracle to interrupt the course of a potentially fatal heart attack, watch a totally occluded vessel open up, see blood flow restored, watch the blood pressure and heart rate normalize, and hear the patients say, "My pain is gone."

*Dr. Crampton dropped by to visit with members of my medical school class as we attended our 45th reunion in Charlottesville in 2016. He looked wonderful and was as dynamic, sharp, and charming as ever. Watching from a slight distance, my wife commented that as we "somewhat older-now" students of medicine stood around him chatting and happily listening to his words, we seemed almost as meek and awed as we must have been so long ago.

Chapter 20: Please, Naught the Yellow Pad!

Another Friday afternoon, I was entering the hospital via the Emergency Ward when the head physician asked if I would do him a tremendous favor. Oh no, I teased, not a Mafia godfather with a massive heart attack who is bound to die, and promises to have the doctor who fails to save him rubbed out? He responded with a huge smile, as if relieved, "No. Worse. An elderly woman with a heart rate of 30 and a son who is a lawyer asking dozens of irrelevant questions, and recording everything on yellow legal size paper." (For the reader, a heart rate of 30 is serious). Apparently another cardiologist who had already been consulted had washed his hands of the situation after 15 minutes of questioning and cross-examination. He declined to take on the case and simply fled the scene.

I introduced myself to the patient and her son, performed a brief examination – enough to know and state simply that this lady could die if we did not promptly put a temporary pacemaker into a vein in the upper leg. I told the son to hold his questions until later, and asked the patient if she would agree to the procedure. I explained that the risks were low of the procedure causing any harm. The risk of doing nothing was very high. She said okay, and we rushed to the catheterization laboratory and put in a temporary pacemaker with, fortunately, no complications. The heart rate was immediately dialed up to 70 beats a minute, and her blood pressure and breathing normalized. Later in the day she received a permanent pacemaker placed under the collarbone by a thoracic surgeon.

The son, who was obviously concerned about his mother, had been suffering from the misconception that his presence and scores of questions while his mother was in unstable, critical condition would improve the quality of care we provided.

Over the next 20 years, the son would often accompany his mother on office visits and make notes. The notes became fewer and he relaxed significantly over time. The pacemaker was checked in the office every three months for almost 11 years. It was programmed to indicate there was only three months of battery life left. As luck would have it however, her pacemaker gave out within one month of the last previous visit. She noticed the difference immediately and came to the emergency room at once. Her heart rate was in the 40s. She was taken to the operating room and the battery was replaced. The son was not overly worried. The patient on the other hand, was angry that the pacemaker did not give the appropriate warning. I could only say that nothing works perfectly and that she received 11 years of excellent functioning, four more years than the average of 7 years. Also, no permanent damage or harm was incurred. She was lucky.

So was the pacemaker company, and so was I. If I had not cheerfully answered 11 years of questions and been totally open and honest about every aspect of her care, a lawsuit from a dissatisfied patient might have resulted with its consequences of years of mental torture, increased fear of future lawsuits, and increased costs for everyone.

The patient lived another 10 years, and died in the hospital of congestive heart failure. We had discussed avoiding a respirator and CPR if there was little hope of reversing the process. Her sons were most attentive, understanding, and at peace with all her decisions. Their final hours with their mother were conducive to closure. I do not think the beginning, the middle, or the end of this story would have been a happy one for anyone had there not been one doctor taking charge and committed in the relationship. What are the chances of that being the case in 2020?

Chapter 21: I Will Not Forget, Annie Roanhorse

It was a typical winter day "On the Res." The sky was its dependable, brilliant blue, and the air was crisp and cool. With the warm sun gleaming, it didn't seem cold at all.

There were the usual 40-60 Navajo adults congregating in the waiting area before 8 AM, speaking Navajo to each other in soft, modulated voices. Most of them had driven 80 to 100 miles over dirt roads to come to town to see an "Anglo" doctor (a foreigner from their vantage point) and, if time permitted, to visit the trading post or general store.

I was waiting in the clinic with one or two other doctors and three nurse interpreters. We were to see all these people before 4 PM, and they would wait patiently for hours to be seen. Regardless of the appointment time they may have been assigned, they almost always arrive before 8 AM since they were up at dawn and had a long, bumpy drive to town and then home again. Most drove pickup trucks which meant that there were usually more people in the back than in the cab.

One of the nurses, Daisy, started the day by ushering a middle-aged woman into an examining room. She introduced me in Navajo and presented me with the chart of Annie Roanhorse. Annie was about 5'4" and weighed 112 pounds. In silhouette, she looked more like me, slender to be kind, scrawny to be truthful, than her compatriots who probably averaged 160 pounds. She was wearing three beautiful velveteen dresses, a squash blossom turquoise necklace, and a Silver conch belt which overlapped two conches in spite of the 3 gowns. She removed the belt and two of the dresses and the interview began. She was 34 years old, married, and had only three children. This fact and her skinny frame caused her to have little clout in the community, and reduced her self-esteem and confidence.

Annie reported being tired all the time and being cold. She kept the two velveteen dresses on top of her while she sat and talked. I leafed through her chart which was at least 3 inches thick, as she had been coming to Shiprock hospital for over 20 years. I could find no record of thyroid function tests. As I circled those on the order sheet, I was pleased to think that I might have found something curable, hypothyroidism. However, I was quick to tell myself that most hypothyroid patients are overweight, not underweight. Nonetheless, there are always exceptions to the rules and the thyroid should be checked. Checking it, however, meant that a blood sample would have to be sent “off the Res” and “comp" money would have to be used. “Comp" meant comprehensive lab test and the money allocated to the PHS for this in July usually ran out by January. Some of the tests ordered by other physicians had been labeled excessive, unnecessary, and wasteful, but at least we were not yet accused of fraud and ordering the tests for profit. We were trying to make a diagnosis and treat the patient appropriately. The tests were not ordered to fill in the blank on a computer screen or follow blindly some algorithm. In short we were doing what we were trained to do decades ago in medical school and residency. When in doubt ask the following question: “What would you do if it was your mother?" Today the question is: “What would the committee or the computer program or the lawyer demand?"

Annie's examination revealed a blood pressure of 100/70, both sitting and standing, and a pulse of 84 which was regular. The thyroid was normal and I found nothing of note. Her weight was unchanged for years.

Her previous laboratory data demonstrated the sodium of 135, the low end of normal, and potassium of five, the high end of normal. Her BUN and hematocrit indicated that she had not been dehydrated or anemic. She had not had menstrual periods for two years. I ordered repeat tests to verify the above values.

I happened to notice that a certain white blood cell called eosinophil was a bit high. This cell was responsible for fighting allergies or infestation with parasites. Annie had not experienced diarrhea or abdominal pain and she was not anemic. Nevertheless, I ordered stool examination for parasites just to be certain.

I was aware that eosinophils may be high in Addison's disease or adrenal insufficiency. I also knew that President Kennedy suffered from Addison's. (While Sen. Lloyd Bentsen of Texas would later state that he had known Jack Kennedy and that Dan Quayle was no Jack Kennedy, I could only note in my brain that I knew what John Kennedy looked like and he bore no resemblance to Annie.)

The point is that I had never ever seen a case of Addison's and so it was at best third on my list of differential diagnoses. I sent Annie home with a bottle of multivitamins ("do no harm!") and a return appointment in three months. I would be waiting for the lab tests but hopefully even the comp lab would be back in one month.

When they came back, there was nothing in the laboratory results of significance. There were no parasites in the stool. The thyroid was normal. Because I was concerned for this patient long after closing time, I reread the chapter on adrenal insufficiency and noted that the borderline blood pressure, sodium, potassium, fatigue, low weight, and eosinophils were all compatible with Addison's. Why, oh why, had I given her a return appointment in three months? It was a "customary" way of doing things.

Annie had no telephone. She lived in a hogan over an hour away. I had her chart pulled and determined where she lived, and asked the community health medic (a high school graduate trained in basic techniques like an Army medic) to locate her and have her come back sooner. She would have to be fasting in order to check another "comp" blood test, a fasting cortisol, and later that day a 4 PM cortisol. Fortunately, Annie was located and agreed to come in for the lab tests. These results would finally confirm the diagnosis of Addison's.

Annie returned yet again within a month after the diagnosis was certain and she was begun on a standard dose of hydrocortisone pills. She began to feel better within a couple of weeks and gained almost 10 pounds a month. When Annie returned three months later (of course) she was almost euphoric for a Navajo. She had gained 30 pounds. Her conch belt no longer overlapped. Her friends and family were rejoicing that she was no longer dead, depressed, bewitched, or hexed. She was her old self. She no longer walked creeping down the hall as though she might stumble or fall over. Her steps were strong, not necessarily a swagger but quick and confident. Her friend had asked her what ceremony she had undergone. She told her friend the "Belagaana" (white person) doctor had cured her. She smiled. The smile said it all... No bonus check has ever felt so fantastic. Thank you, Annie!

For almost 4 decades, I've always noted the eosinophil count.

I knew Annie. I will remember.

Always Look Between the Toes

About forty years ago at a hospital in Ann Arbor,

I was admitting a patient unaware of the need of a safe harbor.

The gentleman was afflicted with cellulitis of the lower

extremity,

Which he attributed to a bite from mosquito or other insect

enemy.

In starting an antibiotic to cure the infection,

I was steering the treatment in the appropriate direction.

The next morning on rounds the astute older attending

Located the place whence the germs were ascending.

Something mundane which everyone knows,

He discovered tinea pedis between the fourth and fifth toes.

A fissure was there, clear as could be,

I learned a good lesson to take home with me.

No matter what someone might suggest or propose,

I will always remember to look 'tween the toes.

Chapter 22: A Dizzying Vertigo Bill

Several studies have estimated that healthcare costs are increased 30 to 40% by legal considerations, including threatened and actual lawsuits. Others disagree but don't actually come up with a number. I cannot be certain myself but I would guess that legal questions likely add at least 20% to healthcare costs. Rather than argue about it, I would ask everyone to agree that whatever the actual number(even if it is 10%), it is simply too much.

As an example of this recurring problem, I would offer the following story. Recently, an 80 year old gentleman awakened with vertigo with the sensation of the room spinning. He had absolutely no other symptoms: no chest pain, no headache, no vomiting, no fever, no abdominal pain, no shortness of breath. It was Sunday morning and his internist was not on call. The covering physician did not know the patient and advised a trip to the Emergency Ward. The gentleman was seen by a nurse and a doctor within 30 minutes, and was sent first for a CT scan of the head and then an MRI of the head. Fortunately, there was no evidence of stroke or brain cancer. There followed a spinal CT of the chest to rule out pulmonary embolism, a CT scan of the chest to rule out lung cancer, and a CT scan of the abdomen to rule out dissecting aneurysm. Of course, there were numerous tests looking for chemical imbalance, anemia, infection, heart attack, and pulmonary embolism. The patient survived this eight hour ordeal (relatively efficient for the number of tests done) and demonstrated no immediate effects of excess radiation. In fact, his vertigo had temporarily subsided at some point. He was discharged home on no medication, a record low I would imagine.????

He visited me two weeks later for routine check of his coronary atherosclerosis following his heart attack five years prior. He was not necessarily astounded so much by his $16,000 EW bill but more by the fact that it had arrived in two weeks. His vertigo had recurred once. I gave him a prescription for meclizine.

The emergency encounter happens multiple times per day in Emergency Wards in the country. The greatest expense for emergency wards is not salaries or technological equipment but the threat of actual lawsuits. As a result, hospitals may take extreme steps to avoid risk of missing a diagnosis.

A potential solution would be to empower a nurse or doctor or physician's assistant at the door of the emergency Ward to truly triage and direct people to less costly alternatives. They would need to be given immunity from lawsuits unless they were determined to be on drugs or grossly derelict. This reform could be mandated by each state legislature on a state-by-state basis. This could be done in a stand-alone piece of legislation or perhaps as part of an effort at broader reform which might include a statewide panel utilizing mediation as an alternative to litigation for medical problems. Of course this would require legislators to look for solutions and not look for campaign contributions from the trial lawyers. Citizens would need to urge their representatives to identify and acknowledge this problem honestly and work with all involved toward fair solutions.

9/5/11

HealthCare Reform

Health Care Reform is presently reborn

And I must admit I am torn

And have a near-fatal dose of scorn

For those who are constantly tooting this horn.

For real cost-cutting steps, I am really forlorn.

There are many who disagree

About the amount of the legal fee

And start climbing up a tree

Insisting that it cannot be.

Let's start with the Emergency Ward.

Take an eighty year-old feeling untoward.

He awakes with his room in a spin,

And no, it was not from gin.

It's Sunday and his doctor's on call,

But he won't want to take the fall.

So off to the ER he goes.

He's examined from his head to his toes.

Then comes the MRIs and CTs times eight

Never mind that the hour is getting quite late.

He must meekly submit to his technological fate.

The good news is that they've ruled out grave ill.

The bad news is he's racked up a SIXTEEN-THOUSAND-

DOLLAR bill !!!

But he should take comfort in knowing

A brain tumor is not yet growing.

Pulmonary embolism and aortic dissection

Will not keep him from voting in the next election.

Heart attack and stroke were not why he awoke.

So what was the problem? Can't anyone say?

Why was the word "vertigo" kept out of play?

Why without meclizine was he sent on his way?

Why in the world did he have an eight-hour stay?

Because triaging and judgement aren't seen as the way

To survive and to practice for another day.

The chance of a lawsuit is feared as abusive

And makes most proposals completely elusive.

The answer requires too much common sense.

Tort reform and mediation are left on the fence.

What is required is a break from the past,

Will the real health reformers step forward at last?

Chapter 23: Ronald Reagan's DRG System, Its Consequences, and Our Need for Other Solutions

This chapter contains my opinions, and my understanding regarding the struggle to change our healthcare system to meet 21st century needs and avoid negative consequences of poorly thought-out steps. It is extremely frustrating to me that payment reforms are packaged in arguments and assumptions that payment reform will drive delivery of better quality care. The struggle to contain costs is an old one now and we still don't have the answers. It is equally frustrating that the answers encompassed in legislation so far and government regulations don't seem to be part of an overall, well designed plan in which someone sees the big picture, knowing the realities of practicing medicine. It seems to have been made more difficult than ever to practice. Who benefits from that?

Going back to the past for lessons about unintended consequences and the need for better thinking, I am amazed at how, for example, few people no matter whether they are patients, doctors, news media, or politicians, even know what the DRG system is, when it was begun, and some unfortunate results. DRG is a price control. It means diagnostic related group. For example, pneumonia may be a DRG or congestive heart failure may be a DRG. Whatever the problem, the hospital is reimbursed a set amount of money regardless if the patient is hospitalized one day or a multitude of days for the same DRG. Medicare and Medicaid reimburse hospitals sometimes even below actual costs anyhow. Payments to hospitals and doctors have been reduced significantly since 1983. Added to that, hospitals are required by law to treat patients in emergency and unstable condition regardless of patient ability to pay at all. A seeming consequence of such price controls, reductions and uncompensated care has been the closure of approximately 500 hospitals nationwide. Was this a planned-for result? If so, why? Who benefits?

Primary care physicians are similarly stressed today. I am told an internist or family practitioner today has trouble clearing an income of $90,000 to $150,000 (before taxes). Often saddled with substantial medical education debt, and with rising costs of everything like other members of society, a young doctor beginning to work cannot likely afford a house in our community, Arlington, Virginia, anymore on that salary. Are they ever likely to earn enough to pay for their children to go to college and graduate school? Thus, is it surprising that only about 1% of United States medical school graduates are planning a career in primary care by the end of their studies? How are the planners lining up incentives to motivate and sustain excellent, dedicated healthcare professionals?

Georgetown University Hospital where I trained in cardiology used to be one of the premier heart programs in our country. The surgeon there, Dr. Hufnagel, implanted the first valve in the aorta decades ago, and the preeminent cardiologist, Dr. Proctor Harvey, trained approximately 8 new cardiologists per year for decades. Today Georgetown University Hospital is owned by a major health system. I understand there is no cardiac catheterization lab, no capability for angioplasty, and no heart surgery at Georgetown Hospital anymore. A patient who happens there with a heart attack would need to be transferred to a facility with the capability of angioplasty or surgery. In a situation where time is critical to the viability of heart muscle and overall survival, this seems counterproductive, if not possibly tragic.

So, who oversees and demands an open, honest, informed discussion of health policy and plans with a view to discovering and vetting choices that might work? Tolerating political gamesmanship and special interests, demonizing different interests for the sake of scoring points will not get the job done. It's not consistent with a successful search for a better system for delivering quality healthcare. Who will inform the public of the questions, and important data from a neutral, objective, analytical, fair viewpoint and not a sensational one?

I am reminded of the movie, Apollo 13. After crippling damage to the Apollo space ship, survival and reentry protocols had to be made for the stranded astronauts, using only what they had available to them in the space capsule. The engineers and flight crew back on earth had to think, devise and test the practicality of different options. The reality of the environment in which the space-stranded pilots had to function was not ignored or put down but instead was fundamental to finding the solution.

So what can we do? Instead of tolerating distraction from the real causes of our problems and high costs, and blaming easier targets, let's insist upon intelligent dialogue, and:

- Think how to reduce Emergency Ward visits by nonemergency patients; empower a triage person to direct patients to less expensive alternatives
- Introduce fair alternative choices to dispute resolution by litigation or its threat to help aggrieved consumers and MDs
- Appoint an independent czar to oversee aspects of the health delivery system, and planning and to

enforce performance expectations for government employees in positions to help or hinder or to commit waste or fraud

- Explore cheaper possibilities for meeting needs for physicians and nurses in needy areas. One might favor a combined college, medical school or other training program with only three years of college, guaranteed participation in primary care with reduced tuition and sufficient salary to be viable. One might even agree ahead of time to the location of the primary care job
- Examine how many physicians and healthcare workers are needed and plan for their training and admission to practice
- Agree that 95% of primary care will be delivered by a physician assistant or advance practice registered nurse

Times are changing for better and worse. Basic science, research, technologies, medications, and therapies are all improving. There are miraculous advances every year. However, these bring with them rising costs. The expanding older population, chronic diseases, extended care facilities, and nursing homes will all contribute to rising costs.

We need to be aware of certain older values and habits that are priceless. Medicine remains a wonderful and uplifting job for everyone from receptionist to technician to social worker to physician's assistant to nurse to doctor to administrator. Computers and technology are important but nothing will ever take the place of the good listener, a familiar face, a kind tone or a patient explanation. After over 40 years of patient care, I am still impressed by the value of a patient seeing the same doctor - "continuity of care." I would strongly recommend that doctors and patients never lose sight of it. Continuity of care has been the cornerstone of medicine for eons. May it continue to be lest we lose for reasons of money, convenience or simply forgetting, the good thing we had.

Chapter 24: Putting the Patient at Ease

A long time ago, I was beginning a procedure, a coronary angiogram and likely angioplasty (balloon opening of a blocked artery to the heart), on an 80-year-old gentleman whom I will call Mr. Thompson. The patient had already received a pill for relaxation but nonetheless he was still somewhat anxious as most all patients are. He was humming a little tune with a fixed gaze toward the ceiling. As I began to numb the area over the femoral artery, I started to hum a song from Showboat:

"Fish gotta swim,

Birds gotta fly,

I'm going to love one man till I die,

Can't help lovin' that man of mine."

The patient joined in, and soon we were jamming, and the technicians were grinning. In the meantime, I had slipped a catheter through a sheath that I had inserted in the femoral artery, and advanced it up to the heart and was ready to take pictures of the arteries. The patient was totally relaxed and stated: "Doc, I know things will be fine when I hear you humming so calmly." I replied that it would be nice if there was a code for relaxation humming as there was for intravenous administration of medication. The angioplasty was completed smoothly, and the patient required no additional sedation.

More recently, a 50-year-old woman we will call Mrs. Jones was awaiting the start of an angiogram. She was trying to relax by joking with the technicians. As I was preparing to numb her upper leg, she challenged my ability to rap. I quickly responded with:

"So you think that I can't rap

Well just go ahead and yap

I'll quickly numb your lap

Then your arteries I will map

Feel free to take a nap!"

Knowing the patient's personality from previous visits and being able to respond on the same plane, allowed the patient to relax to a greater degree and more safely than with intravenous "controlled substances."

As time goes by, there are fewer single physician practices and many more large group practices, so there is less chance of getting to know each patient and forming a relationship. This results in the patient's being more anxious and the doctors being more tense. This in turn creates conditions where imperfect outcomes are more likely to result in animosity and even lawsuits. Continuity of care should at the very least include meeting with the physician performing the procedure ahead of time so that there is the opportunity, however brief, of establishing some familiarity with the patient.

Chapter 25: How Not to Choose a Doctor

A few years ago, an elderly lady began her routine visit for high blood pressure by asking if I would listen to her latest experience. She had traveled to a well reputed university hospital for a cataract operation. She had interacted through the Internet, was given an appointment for surgery, and reportedly never saw the ophthalmologist. She states that she was prepped and was lying on the table when the doctor came into the OR and put on his gown and gloves. At that point, she relates that she coughed once. The doctor did not introduce himself but simply pulled off his gloves, told the nurse to reschedule the patient, and left. She dressed, went home, and waited. No one had called her in the two weeks that followed. Part of what mattered is the patient's perception of what had happened.

I advised her not to go back to that institution or doctor. There are many personable, courteous, and competent physicians located locally. The best way to find a good physician is not by surfing the web or googling a famous institution. I would bet that very few people if any select their hairdresser from the Internet. The best route for choosing a doctor is to check with your primary care physician or any physician whom you trust, or perhaps ask a friend who has already had their procedure. I would advise against relying solely on hospital referral lists; they may not be more than lists of physicians employed by that hospital or lists of members of the independent medical staff.

Chapter 26: INH: The Cure

In 1954 the number one killer in the US and the world was Tuberculosis (TB). Almost every state had a number of TB sanatoria and they were full of dying, debilitated, contagious people who were hoping that mountain air and changing environment would be the cure. It is virtually impossible for Americans born after WWII to grasp how deadly and rapacious the disease was, taking its toll among so many young people who had been in the prime of their lives.

Every hospital admission was screened for TB with the PPD skin test. Then isoniazid was developed (INH). A plan was formed to try this new medicine on the Navajo reservation where the rate of infection was over 550%. A team of physicians was organized from Cornell Medical School – New York Hospital to institute a screening and treatment program at Many Farms, close to Canyon de Chelly (pronounced "Shay") in Arizona. One of the physicians involved in the project was Jerry Mandel, who would later become my medical school advisor and head of infectious diseases at the University of Virginia Medical School.

INH worked. It was nothing short of a miracle. Most cases of TB were improved and cured as long as people were closely monitored and encouraged to stick with the program for two years. Contacts or people exposed were given INH for one year as a preventive if their TB skin test was positive. No one was reported to die from the medicine. In spite of the fact that it was later determined that over 50% of patients had changes in their liver tests that were 10 times normal, the medication was not stopped. Today one rarely hears about routine TB except perhaps in immigrants. Drug-resistant TB has become a problem in those who do not stick to the program or whose immune systems are weakened by AIDS or cancer. Dr. Paul Farmer has dedicated himself to the treatment of drug-resistant TB worldwide and has convinced the makers of several little-used drugs to provide these agents at low cost. What a difference one person can make!

Through Dr. Mandel's work setting up a program whereby a third or fourth year University of Virginia medical student could spend two months on the Navajo reservation, I eventually spent two months in Fort Defiance in 1970 and later volunteered for two more years at Shiprock from 1973 to 1975. I was quite active in the program of screening, reviewing chest x-rays, and treating TB.

While I was on call one night, a 36-year-old man, married, a father of four, was transferred from an outlying clinic with the referring physician presuming the complaint of *vomiting* up blood.(Actually, the patient spoke no English and was interviewed through interpreters. The interpreter told the referring physician the patient said he was *coughing* up blood.) The referring physician had passed an NG tube into the stomach where he found fresh blood. In addition, the chest x-ray was negative. Also, the patient was not coughing. He seemed fine. I found him a bed in the children's ward, at the end of the hall, in an isolation room and gave him antacids in case he had a stomach ulcer. I ordered sputum for TB (AFB acid fast bacillus), but he still wasn't coughing.

I went to bed but was awakened two hours later because the man was frantically running around the room coughing blood onto the walls. I stayed with him for 30 minutes until the coughing stopped. I gave him some medicine for anxiety and ordered INH. I scooped up some of the clotted blood to go to the lab for culture, which might take a month for results. The next day I passed him along to another physician with the presumed diagnosis that he had TB even though his chest x-ray was still normal and he was no longer coughing.

When I returned several weeks later, I was devastated to learn that the man had died. He had had another coughing fit with copious clumps of blood which obstructed his breathing. I am still saddened and wonder what else could have been done. He would have had to be transferred to a hospital in Albuquerque two hundred or more miles away.

I can't imagine the sorrow his wife and children suffered and may still be suffering. Fortunately, relatively few people die of TB anymore. The development of multiple medications for TB has been a miracle and a blessing. No doubt about it.

Chapter 27: Aunt Minnie: A Variation on The Theme

For over 10 years from 2000 to 2011, I was a member of a voluntary group of doctors, nurses, optometrists, physical therapists, and lay citizens who traveled to Honduras for one week each year. The group has performed over 70 operations per week, examined and dispensed medicines to over 4000 people, and provided prescription eyeglasses to 2500 individuals. Other group members worked in more remote villages to provide clean, running water off the mountains with sinks and toilets. An orphanage on a mountaintop run by two diminutive nuns managing 15 children received baking utensils, a stove, bread-making instructions, and a cow. The brigade was founded by Dr. Barry Byer in connection with his local church and a group named Crosslink.

On my first trip to Honduras in 2000, I had finished seeing a patient and was waiting for another to be brought to me when I saw a young girl whom I will call Alma, standing with her mother and younger brother. The girl's eyes were bulging outward and one could see the white of her eyes all the way around the brown iris. I brought Alma and her family to my interview area and immediately started to examine her and ask questions. She had not slept through the night for three years. She wet her bed every night. She was nervous, sweaty, had diarrhea, and felt her heart beating fast all the time. Her pulse was 140 and her hands trembled. Her thyroid was very much enlarged. She clearly had Graves' disease with an overactive thyroid. The only medicine that we had that might be helpful was a beta blocker named atenolol which counteracts adrenaline and slows down the pulse and the tremors, and reduces the anxiety. On the spot, I gave her 100 mg, with a plastic bag of 30 more to take home.

Alma returned the next day to report that she had slept through the night and felt a zillion (*no se como se dice en Espanol*) times better. The heart rate was 90 and there was no tremor. I introduced her and her family to one of the Honduran army officers on the base where we were located and also to the First Lady of Honduras, Mary Flores, who visited every day. Arrangements were made to have Alma treated by an endocrinologist in Tegucigalpa, the capital. I also introduced Alma to one of the physicians whom I had surmised as having Grave's Disease 10 years earlier across an auditorium. It was comforting to her and her mother to see someone who had recovered from hyperthyroidism and who was totally functional and not too unattractive (*chiste*).

Recognizing from afar that Alma's eyes reflected a major problem is another example of how knowing Aunt Minnie and being on the lookout for her may save time and avoid errors.

Chapter 28: Couples: One

One of the privileges of my practice has been the number of couples who have come to my office for decades. Some of them began their visits by having one of them come alone and check out the office. Others first came together. Most of them choose to stay in the examining room together. They enjoy being together and do not wish to be separated. It is very sweet. Today one would say it is pretty cool. They help each other relax, correct portions of the history (medications, operations, dates of things etc.), and ask appropriate questions. After they leave, they remember instructions and explanations better. The entire arrangement is much more pleasant and more effective. It's almost like a party but without food or drink.

One such couple was particularly happy together and I will call them the Sunshines. They were native to Virginia, married in their 20s, and lived together for 60 years. They were both relatively small, soft spoken, pleasant, and most attentive to each other's needs. They weathered heart attacks, angioplasties, and the effects of aging gracefully and without complaint. Around age 80, Mrs. Sunshine developed severe congestive heart failure and died. Her husband was extremely sad and lonely without his loving mate. He continued to come to the office for a few years but was simply not happy. (One could say that he was depressed but with good reason. Medication was not the answer.)

Then one visit he began the conversation with a broad smile and said he had some wonderful news that might surprise me. "I'm getting married!" he announced with a booming joyful voice. He explained that he had accidentally run into his high school sweetheart who was also widowed and that they had decided to spend their remaining years together. Mrs. Sweet 16 had revived Mr. Sunshine. They remained devoted bosom buddies for years. Mr. Sunshine passed on peacefully in his sleep in his home of 70 years. Thank you for the memories and for teaching me that keeping spouses together in the office is often more user-friendly, and beneficial.

Chapter 29: Couples: Take Two

Another couple who started to come to my office early on I will call the Steeles. They were approximate 50 years old and were committed to each other and to their children, two of whom were mentally challenged. Although they enjoyed a good joke, they were most interested in accurate diagnosis, effective treatment, availability of their physician, and straight talk. They both were overweight, under active, and had multiple coronary risk factors including high blood pressure, elevated cholesterol and latent diabetes. Today they would be categorized as having metabolic syndrome.

Over time they both developed severe coronary artery atherosclerosis and required balloon angioplasties. After 25 years of intense care, Mr. Steele died of congestive heart failure. The children became obese, smoked, did not exercise, and developed their own cardiac conditions. Mrs. Steele continue to be a bulwark of strength, making sure her children were monitored and cared for. She suffered from arthritis and she lived on into her late 90s. She was satisfied that her children would receive good care. On every visit, she would make sure to ask for assurance that I was not about to retire. This, of course, was a form of compliment.

Her greatest concern was that she would pass out, be resuscitated, be placed on a respirator, given the feeding tube and IV fluids and kept alive with miniscule hope of recovery. She filled out a living will. She asked if I would take her off a respirator and discontinue everything if the situation was such that she would not be able to speak, communicate, move around, or feed herself. Since she only trusted me to carry out her wishes, she remained in Arlington and instructed her helpers to take her to Arlington hospital (now Virginia Hospital Center) if she was sick. She named me as her medical power of attorney. Happily, she passed away in her sleep at home, just as she had planned. I am most grateful for the gift she gave me: absolute trust.

Chapter 30: Living Will, a.k.a." Right to Die"

My wife is a wonderful person and I try desperately not to hold it against her that she is a lawyer. She is active in an impressive voluntary group called the Virginia Bar Association (VBA), which advises the Legislature, runs CLE programs, community service projects, and provides pro bono services. She does not know how to say "no." Years ago, she was on three PTA-type organizations simultaneously, a quasi-triple agent.

10 years ago, she set up a community education program with a young VBA lawyer at the Alexandria courthouse to teach citizens about the living will law in Virginia and help people fill out their own forms. She had snookered her VBA friend - a wonderful lawyer named Bob McAllister - into participating, and I was informed that if I wanted supper I had best "volunteer" too. So I did. Reluctantly!

There were eight people in the audience when the program started. Two were asleep and three others later excused themselves to use the facilities. The teacher-student ratio was the highest ever in the state as reported in the local Virginia Gazette. (The volunteers' names were withheld upon my request and I surmise that there would be triple the number of phone calls and requests.) My wife says I exaggerate this story. (He does – grossly! Ed.)

Bob, who is an excellent attorney, opened the program with some general remarks such as, "None of us is getting any younger." He was just getting to the meat of his talk when a 70-ish white-haired lady raised her hand and called out, "May I ask a question?" Bob hesitated, stepped backward, and said "Yes, I guess so." What he probably wanted to say was, "How can you have a question when I haven't even started yet?" The lady proceeded to relate an episode from five years before involving her mother having a heart attack and being in a coma. A doctor had called this woman to inform her that her mother was unlikely to recover but that he could perform an experimental procedure (she could not remember what it was called) that might save her life. The doctor asked if the patient would ever consent to such a procedure or whether the daughter would consent. The daughter stated emphatically that she knew her mother would absolutely refuse such a procedure but that she herself would be strongly in favor of it. She instructed the doctor to proceed, which he did. Four days later the mother regained consciousness and she lived three more years. The lady wanted to know what Bob thought of this scenario.

Bob probably was wondering about assault and battery charges, whether there was a psychiatrist in the room, or about paging himself out of the meeting. He appeared to be speechless, a state I wished my lawyer wife would slip into occasionally. I volunteered to answer the lady's question. "Ma'am, first I would like to ask you how your mother felt when she awakened and was informed of what had transpired." She replied that her mother was furious, and stated she wished nothing had been done. As far as her mother was concerned she had experienced a most peaceful and timely death.

I addressed the audience (all three of the semiconscious attendees) and told them that the situation was perfect. I did. I said that this lady provided the clearest example of whom not to pick for your medical power of attorney. She was obviously a very kind, caring, and rational individual. However, this lady had not carried out her mother's wishes. The role of the medical power of attorney is to try to judge what the patient would wish and inform the doctor and not introduce her own wishes.

At that point I turned to Bob and suggested that he continue his presentation. He did. He spoke eloquently and ended to a nice round of applause. I added for those present that there is an inherent contradiction in our system. When asked, 99% of my patients state that they want to die in their sleep in their own bed at home. However, 99% of their relatives respond that they do not want their loved ones dying at home; they prefer for them to die in the hospital or in a nursing home or at hospice. There is an overwhelming tendency not to discuss end-of-life plans or simply to ignore them.

Communication with the medical power of attorney, family members, other relatives, and even neighbors might result in the desired care that the patient has wished for, by starting the living will process in the first place. It might. It might even reduce the gigantic medical bill at the end of life at which time it is estimated that a large chunk of the healthcare dollar (estimated at 70% in some articles) is used by 10% of the population in the last six months of life.

Chapter 31: Trust - Part One; Deep

There was a lady of around 60 years of age whom I will call Mrs. No Heme. I met her as she entered the hospital with unstable angina. She had new onset severe chest discomfort at rest and with minimal exertion including going poop. Her coronary angiogram demonstrated severely obstructed coronary arteries (95 to 98% occlusions) involving all three branches. This is called triple vessel coronary artery disease and it merits a triple coronary bypass operation. The cardiac surgeon was consulted, explained the procedure to her and its risks, and was about to call and schedule the procedure immediately. But the lady had a question that he had never heard which stopped him short.

The lady simply asked the surgeon if he would let her bleed to death. His response was something she did not want to hear. He replied, " Of course not." She explained that she was either a Seventh-day Adventist or a Christian scientist. I can't recall which. In any event she did not believe in receiving blood transfusions, but she would submit to the operation if the surgeon would promise not to give her a blood transfusion. The surgeon said that he could not in good conscience promise that. Hence, the operation did not take place.

She remained in the hospital for three weeks. She was mildly anemic and received ERYTHROPOETIN injections but her blood count remained unchanged. She was still having rest and exertional pain, in bed and in the bathroom, in spite of maximal medical treatment. She was headed toward a massive heart attack and likely death.

She finally asked me if I could balloon her arteries. I told her that each blockage carried a risk of 1 to 2% of heart attack or death, and that she might experience kidney failure, and arrhythmia, and sudden death. I said I would do it if she was determined to abide by her religious beliefs and not consent to the surgery. She asked if I would let her die if she bled out. I told her that I had never had anyone die from a procedure, that I had no intention of "letting her die," that I would use lactated ringers as was used in Vietnam and have a surgeon stop the bleeding if necessary; I would honor her wishes not to give her blood. However I wanted her husband, her minister, and any significant friend to confer with her and write down their conviction about her avoiding blood products.

The procedure was scheduled for the next day. The consent form included the exclusion of blood transfusion. I was more concerned about the risk of heart attack and death than of bleeding. After all, this was before the time of stents; a sudden collapse of an artery after deflating the balloon was not uncommon.

The procedure was a success. The balloon fit all three vessels and all three blockages disappeared from sight with two brief inflations each. The total time it took was 40 min. Mrs. No Heme experienced no pain and there was no bleeding. She went home the next day and did not experience any recurrences of her pain. Her prayers were answered regarding no blood products. My prayers were answered with a living, functionally intact patient. Hallelujah!

Chapter 32: Trust Extended Over Space and Time

No one enjoys getting sick while traveling. It is an uncomfortable situation meeting new doctors and entering unfamiliar emergency wards in hospitals when you had expected to be doing something else. Fear and doubt are constantly present. Quite simply, it's scary.

Once a month or more I receive an urgent long-distance phone call from a physician who is caring for a patient of mine. The patient usually has some non-cardiac problem which requires a procedure but the patient is reluctant to accept the word of an unfamiliar physician. The patient insists that the doctor call me to verify and reassure them. If the patient cannot come to the phone I generally tell the doctor to say that we have spoken and everything seems to be appropriate. I will have reviewed the charts and concluded that the risk of a heart attack should be low so they should do well. I may advise the physician to continue a medicine, such as a beta blocker, intravenously if the patient is unable to eat or swallow. The patient always thanks me for taking the phone call, reassuring them and the physician.

Some time ago, I was examining the patient in my office when my nurse knocked on the door and said there was an emergency phone call from North Carolina. I excused myself to take the call. I was surprised to hear from the doctor that an 80-year-old patient of mine whom we may call Mr. Doubtfire was in an emergency ward with severe right lower quadrant abdominal pain, fever, elevated WBC, and vomiting. The physician explained that there was a high likelihood of appendicitis and the longer they put off surgery the greater the chance of rupture.

The patient would normally have been very agreeable but something didn't seem right. The doctor handed the phone to the patient and I told him that he really had no choice and the sooner he consented to the operation the better, even if it turned out not to be appendicitis. He thanked me profusely and said he would immediately give his okay. He said all he really needed was to hear the sound of my voice. A month later when Mr. Doubtfire visited my office, he again thanked me and stated how appreciative he was. It was appendicitis as suspected.

It cannot be stated too often that the benefits of continuity of care are vast and that the worth cannot be tabulated in dollars. This may be lost forever if larger and larger groups are created and patients see a different healthcare provider each visit.

Chapter 33: Aunt Minerva to Aunt Minnie

During the end of my internship in Ann Arbor, I was rotating through the walk-in clinic at the University hospital. I had seen a 65-year-old lady who had presented with cough, fever and shortness of breath for two days; her throat was normal. She had no swollen glands. She could not produce phlegm. Her lungs were clear. She was rotund but that was not the issue. She voiced no other complaints. I treated her with an antibiotic and a decongestant, and told her to call if she was not better in two days. I moved on to the next room and what seemed like an endless line of patients.

The next day, the lady returned now coughing up phlegm. She was seen by Dr. Jeff Strumpf, my supervising resident, who read my note and called me into the room, and asked if I recognized the patient. I said that I did. He asked what else did I see. I replied that she was overweight, but I had no idea what he was getting at. He had me examine her skin - it was coarse. He had me check her thyroid. It was perhaps mildly enlarged but hard to discern. Then he asked me to check her eyebrows; the outside third was missing. He instructed me to ask the patient how she was doing. She replied, "Not better" in a deep voice. Jeff said, "This is a classic case of hypothyroidism (underactive thyroid)." The light went on in my head immediately. I had just been introduced to another Aunt Minnie.

I had never yet seen a patient with hypothyroidism, and so I only knew her as Aunt Minerva - a distant relative, actually a stranger. From that moment on I have tried to observe the whole patient and to consider the diagnosis of hypothyroidism in many people, especially those who are overweight.

Over the years, I have had the good fortune to be associated with a multitude of excellent physicians. I have been able to have lunch at Arlington Hospital in the designated room for doctors and I've been able to discuss specific cases and general concerns. Repeatedly, I have inquired about the standard lab test "normals" for hypothyroidism but was only told that they were under discussion.

Finally, in 2005 Dr. Bob Santangelo, an Endocrinologist, told me that my concerns were well-founded and that in fact there was a committee that was trying to reach an agreement on correcting the previously accepted upper limit of normal of "TSH." He referred me to Dr. Wartofsky at the Washington Hospital Center who is a recognized expert on hypothyroidism. Besides speaking to Dr. Wartofsky by phone, I was also able to read his opinion in a journal article published that year in 2005.

The thyroid is like the foreman of an automobile factory with multiple divisions. It is up to the foreman to send messages to all the other divisions on how fast they should do their jobs. The foreman, the thyroid, sets the idle for every organ of the body. Above the foreman sits the CEO, in this case the pituitary, who monitors what kind of job the thyroid is doing. If the thyroid is underactive, the pituitary sends more messages telling it to turn out more thyroid hormone. The messages are called thyroid stimulating hormone, TSH, so the body has what is called a negative feedback system or a kind of thermostat. If the thyroid produces too much thyroid hormone (T-3 or T4), then the pituitary decreases or shuts off the amount of TSH that is produced.

The laboratory listed the normal TSH as .4 to 5.5 for decades; however, this is apparently intentionally incorrect.

Somehow it was decided years ago that it would be wise to set a high threshold of normal in order to prevent the undue use or abuse of thyroid hormone medication for weight reduction. There is still disagreement as to what to list as normal. Many labs have reduced the upper limit of TSH (the threshold for treatment) from 5.5 down to 4.5. In reality the normal upper limit is closer to 1.5 to 2.5. Most endocrinologists that I have spoken to are comfortable initiating treatment if the TSH is above 3.

A different area of concern is not the threshold for beginning treatment but the goal. The goal is a value of the TSH from 1 to 1.5. But again, there is disagreement among the experts. There is concern that an irregular heart rhythm, or osteoporosis may be induced if treatment is begun abruptly and with too high a dose of thyroid hormone (levothyroxine or brand name Synthroid). Hence it is wise to initiate treatment at 25 mcg per day and increase the dose by 25 mcg every three weeks until the TSH is 1 to 1.5. This is a general guideline recommended to me and so far, it has been extremely effective and very safe with no evidence of arrhythmia or osteoporosis as of yet. In general, however it is always true that the numbers are only a guideline and that one should treat the patient as a whole, on an individual basis.

There are many areas affected by an underactive thyroid. First of all, obesity or simply being overweight has numerous related problems besides decreased mobility - tendency to fall, diabetes, metabolic syndrome, increased risk of heart attack and stroke, atherosclerosis, and Alzheimer's disease.

Abnormal total cholesterol, triglycerides, good cholesterol, and bad cholesterol may all be influenced by an underactive thyroid. Treatment significantly improves the lipid profile and reduces the need for other medicines. Everyone with abnormal lipid should have their TSH tested.

A third area of concern is a slow heartbeat. Some patients have had heart rates as low as 30 beats a minute. Consideration of a permanent pacemaker is appropriate at a heart rate of 46 or less. With treatment of hypothyroidism, some pacemakers might possibly be avoided or postponed. Most people who do not exercise enough have a heart rate above 70 BPM. If someone says that they do not exercise at all and yet their heart rate is 60 or less, the thyroid should be evaluated.

A fourth area of concern is weakness of the heart muscle, sometimes labeled a cardiomyopathy (CM). This may sometimes be attributed to alcohol, coronary atherosclerosis, a virus, postpartum, or unknown cause. I have seen a number of individuals who have been told that the cause is unknown and that their congestive heart failure is worsening. Not only may the TSH be above three but there are cases where the TSH is normal and the total T3 is low - less than .1. Thyroid hormone treatment has resulted in improved function and in some cases normalization of the ejection fraction (the amount of blood pumped out of the pumping chamber each beat) on echocardiography.

Fifth, there is a certain percentage of patients who are diagnosed with depression who are hypothyroid. They may never have had their TSH checked or due to the incorrect level of normal listed they may go undiagnosed as being hypothyroid. Some whom I have treated for their cardiac condition of heart failure or bradycardia have been able to reduce their medication or get off of their antidepressant medication with the guidance of their psychiatrist.

Sixth, anemia may result from a number of causes. Sometimes, especially in menstruating women, iron deficiency may be the cause. In this situation the red blood cells are small in diameter (MCV less than 80). In other cases the red blood cells are large (MCV above 98) and there is a deficiency of vitamin B12 or folic acid or the presence of alcoholism or underactive thyroid. Many times since the thyroid is considered normal according to the erroneous lab TSH upper limit of normal the patient is labeled as anemia of unknown etiology. In treating their low HDL or congestive heart failure with the lowest dose of thyroid hormone 25 mcg a number of people have had their anemia resolved.

The list of other symptoms or signs possibly caused by an underactive thyroid is lengthy: fatigue, decreased energy, difficulty sleeping, waking up tired, feeling cold, cold hands and feet, decreased focus, forgetfulness, memory loss, coarse or dry skin, constipation, hair loss, loss of outer third of eyebrows, menstrual irregularities, decreased libido(decreased testosterone), edema, hoarse or deep voice decreased reflexes.

At some point the committee reviewing this issue will change the normal TSH of .4 to 4 to a more appropriate guideline of .4 to 3 or perhaps 2.5, but this will not happen soon. In the meantime, doctors and patients should keep an eye out for Aunt Minerva and consider hypothyroidism in their differential diagnoses for a number of complaints and abnormal findings.

Chapter 34: Relationships, Illness and Death

Being open to any kind of reimbursement plan has introduced me to many different patients and their cultures. One of the common occurrences over the years is to see a child accompany and translate for their parent and grandparent from Vietnam or El Salvador or Ethiopia or Afghanistan. The respect shown to their elders is heartwarming. It is also noteworthy that babies of immigrants are less stimulated and generally ignored during an office visit. There seems to be less crying and fussiness. I wonder if there is a connection.

I have now been fortunate to meet members of families with grandparents, parents and children. Sometimes diagnosing ailments that are genetic or familial is much easier and explaining the need for a medicine is simpler because someone in the family has already talked about their own problem. A condition like mitral valve prolapse may be quite worrisome until one learns that grandma or mom both have it. Then the headaches, chest pain, palpitations, dizziness, migraines and anxiety are lessened significantly. I also have the patient and perhaps the parents listen for the click and murmur of mitral valve prolapse with my stethoscope while the patient is standing. This reduces the chance of the patient being confused by another healthcare provider who has a suboptimal stethoscope or does not listen with the patient standing and tells the patient he or she does not have mitral valve prolapse. Most of the time the findings can be demonstrated even though they may be intermittent. In addition, medication and exercise reduce the loudness of the murmur further.

It is worth repeating that many issues, including end of life decisions are easier for everyone when the doctor, the decision-maker and the rest of the family know each other. It is not hard to feel sad and demonstrate sadness when someone you have taken care of for a decade or four is dying. In days of yore the General Practitioner visited the dying patient at home or in the hospital probably multiple times in spite of there being "little that could be done." The job description included palliation, including morphine, consoling, and helping folks grieve. The four stages of dying may not have been clearly delineated on paper until Kubler-Ross wrote On Death and Dying, but they were undoubtedly understood by the majority of physicians. Now we seem to need a booklet, a course, or an app.

3/27/09

⌈!!G□ AL!!⌉

The clock is ticking.
The end is near,
But do not forget,
To be of joy and good cheer.

The game is known.
We are all meant to die.
So let us not bemoan.
There is no need to cry.

Life is so short,
But ever so sweet.
Don't build a big fort
Or look down at your feet.

It's not about you,
Or the life that we live.
It's all about others
And what you can give.

Family is first,
So that's where you start.
Take care of their thirst,
Before you depart.

Friends are forever.

They'll understand.
This last endeavor
Is not what you planned.

Community ties run deep and far.
Don't let them lose track of the brotherhood's star.
Fraternities provide nurture and love,
Spreading the message of peace, like a dove.

Life, like a run,
down the field,
toward a goal,
has zigs
and zags.
Sometimes the ball hits the pole.

When time has expired,
What one hopes to remember
Is slipping the ball past
The lone,
last defender

The assemblage erupts with a noise that is din-ish,
"Thank goodness" they say.
Such a glorious finish!

6/2/12

One Day: A Centenarian

Nighttime comes ever so slowly.
The prospect of peace seems ever so holy.
The body and mind struggle each day
Wondering how much more must they pay.

The tolls weren't so onerous when youth shared the task.
The penance was cleansing once the challenge had passed.
With ten decades of caring and wearing so well,
Now all of a sudden it's turned into hell.

The pain is present from dawn to dusk.
The smell all around me has turned to musk.
A spritz of perfume, a brief distraction,
Nothing prolonged, no grand satisfaction.

The pills no longer seem to dull the pain,
But only add confusion to the strain on the brain,
Letters and calls from family and friends,
Increase in number as I near the end.

What can I say as I lay chained to my bed
With someone to change me and help me get fed?
I have been loved by many, it's true.
Eighteen great-grandchildren have filled out my crew.

But the ship is past saving.
There's nothing to do.

Dry rot and rust,
paint and polish can't renew.

The parts will eventually be returned to their Maker.
They'll be used to create a cute little faker,
A baby with eyes maybe blue or brown
And whose smell is like perfume spread all around.

So this is the way of the World we know.
Nature and nurture determine the show.
The time is nearing to say "So long."
When the spirit has left me, don't beat on the gong.

Please climb up the tower and ring every bell.
Gather together and stories do tell.
Spreading joy and love across this great land,
For life and living are truly quite grand.

Chapter 35: Then and Now: Teaching Kindness and Compassion

Through the years and as indicated previously, I have had the privilege of caring for people from different countries. In the 1970s and 1980s there were numbers from Vietnam. In the 1980s and 1990s there were refugees from Afghanistan, Cambodia and Ethiopia to name a few. Uniformly they have seemed very thankful to be here in America in spite of the fact that they were almost always poor. Some already had Medicaid when I first saw them. Most had nothing. Some insisted on paying $10.00 per month (is this the opposite of Boutique Medicine?). Many I saw for free. So did quite a number of other physicians in our medical community.

My father was a pediatrician in Manhattan, affiliated with Cornell Medical Center, and for a time Chief of Pediatrics at Memorial Sloan-Kettering. He would occasionally tell me about poor families he had treated in Florida where he was stationed during WWII. There were people who were perennially poor in New York City, children of alcoholics who never paid, foreigners attached to the United Nations, and of course 50-100 medical residents or medical students with children. He took care of these people essentially for free. He never sent out a bill collector when there was a recession. He maintained the same low office visit fee from 1945 to 1963. He refused to split up the DPT vaccine so he could have 3 separate charges.

He never owned a home but rented an apartment in NYC. To him the American Dream did not involve owning a home. The American Dream to him was freedom from debt. He purchased a Ford with cash and a trade in every 2 years, buying the car from a friend's dealership in the North Country, timing the purchase with his annual trek back to his birthplace there. He owed no one any money and in fact financed the education of various relatives besides his own 3 sons'. He also made house calls. (Sometimes, at night, he had me sit in the car, which was double parked, to make sure the police did not give him a ticket.)

My grandfather in law, John White, graduated from Columbia P&S (for Physicians and Surgeons), having skipped college altogether. He set up practice on 46th Street and 8th Avenue in his home in NYC. During the 1918 flu epidemic, after seeing his patient on a house call, he would make his way from the floor where the patient had called for him up to the top floor, stopping to see everyone whom he could, then cross over the roof to the next building, working his way back down to the street. He said people had left their apartment doors open asking, calling out for help – anyone for help.

He was well known to the theater people. He often took money out of his pocket, literally, so that a cash-strapped patient could buy the medicine he was prescribing. When I met him he was 90 years old and in a nursing home where he was still offering advice when asked by his fellow residents. His mind remained unusually sharp.

I grew up on 88th Street on the 10th floor of an apartment building. The apartment next to ours was occupied by Dr. Haas and his family. Dr. Haas had fled Munich in 1936. He was a GP who performed surgery. He was a soft-spoken, pleasant, cheerful gentleman who exuded courtesy and concern. He remained in practice until he was 90 years old (!) dedicated to his patients and his profession.

So much has changed. Not as many doctors see patients for free even though Medicaid itself reimburses very little and might feel like free to some. Medicare does not pay appropriately so that many physicians do not accept Medicare patients anymore. Doctors like other folks prefer set hours and don't like to be rushed. Office practices follow models and advice set by medical business consultants. They don't necessarily try to accommodate patients with urgent problems but partly for legal purposes, the patient may be advised to go straight to the ER. Since remuneration is low and time is now so important, many physicians have even stopped seeing their patients when they are admitted to the hospital. Hospital based doctors now care for most of the patients there.

Stranger still is the concern that hospitals have regarding patient satisfaction about such items as food, bedding, and comfort of visitors. These areas are of increasing importance due to patient satisfaction polls and rankings in a national magazine. It is a marketing issue. Money and time are being spent on teaching medical residents how to smile, initiate physical contact, establish eye contact and maintaining distance from the patient. There will at some point be an app on kindness and compassion. Characteristics that used to be expected as an aspect of professionalism and assumed to be already present in medical school applicants are perhaps not anymore. I don't know exactly why.

Back in the 1950s and 1960s in "cold," unfeeling New York City, we were taught to stop what we were doing and help a blind person cross the street. We were taught to hold a door for someone and to give up our seat on a bus or subway for an elderly person. Clearly these courtesies are not being taught the same in today's school and homes. Don't we need to emphasize core values starting at an early age? I think the best way is to teach community concern and service with the parents leading the way, the earlier the better.

Chapter 36: Chance Encounter

One day around 2 pm, I was walking through the ER on my way into the hospital when I was waved down by one of the young physicians. (In retrospect, my error was taking that shortcut from office to patient floors - or else I was speeding, i.e., simply walking too fast.) In any event, I was asked if I could give an opinion on a patient that was a bit of a puzzle. I said I would be happy to help. (Of course, I was running late, but no matter.)

The doctor said he was evaluating a 45-year-old man with a funny-looking EKG and a very strange kind of chest pain.

I perused the EKG for less than 30 seconds and remarked as how there were Q waves, downward deflections in two leads, V1 and V2, which suggested that a heart attack had occurred in the past or was actually occurring at the present. There were also ST elevations in the same leads, which strongly suggested the heart attack was taking place right then or within the past few hours. The other ten leads of the EKG were totally normal.

The patient was very pleasant, full of smiles, and supposedly not having chest pain at that moment. I say "supposedly" because the majority of patients with chest pain who have had some improvement in their symptoms (perhaps from the administration of oxygen) deny that they are in pain. Doctors and nurses should be asking: "Does your chest feel normal?" Many times the answer is "no." There is still some residual tightness or pressure but not "pain" or anything that the patient can't endure. The patient is missing the point and so is the health care provider.

If the patient is still having symptoms and their blood pressure is normal or high, then giving a sublingual (under the tongue) nitroglycerin (NTG SL) may result in the complete resolution of symptoms within a few minutes. The patient may be able to say "yes" in response to the question "does your chest now feel totally normal?" This affirms that the symptoms are most likely from the heart and due to a reduction of blood flow (ischemia) and that the NTG has improved blood flow quickly and has reduced the blood pressure and the work of the heart.

Sometimes the ER doctor will apply nitroglycerine paste. This is glopped on the skin (not smeared) and is poorly, slowly, and not uniformly absorbed. There is not the same diagnostic effect nor is there the delivery of a therapeutic amount of medication.

Our patient, whom we will call Mr. Dear, had the onset of severe chest pain 4 days earlier. The pain involved the entire chest, was generally sharp, and resolved only when he went running. The description in no way resembled the pain of heart pain, either angina (temporary reversible heart ischemia) or a heart attack (permanent damage).

However, after he received a NTG SL under the tongue, his symptoms (which were actually "pressure," not pain) resolved within 2 minutes. I informed him that he should not go home, that he needed various medications immediately, and that he should have an angiogram to see if there was a blockage of the coronary arteries.

At that moment, the ER doctor entered to report that the troponin (a blood test for heart muscle) was abnormal, confirming that he was in the middle of a heart attack. Some damage had already occurred. Some may have occurred 4 days earlier. However, a lot more could occur if the blocked artery was not opened up. His chance of death could be reduced from approximately 15% to 4% with a balloon angioplasty or stent. From the EKG one could judge that the blockage involved the left main or proximal LAD: the so called "widow-maker" lesion.

The patient was given a bolus of heparin, an aspirin 81 mg and Plavix 75 mg 4 tablets to reduce blood clotting at the site of the blockage. He was also placed on IV (intravenous) NTG to lower the systolic BP to 110 mm Hg and IV metoprolol (a beta blocker that counteracts adrenaline) to reduce the heart rate to approximately 60 beats per minute (BPM). He was taken to the catheterization laboratory within 15 minutes. Coronary angiography (X ray pictures of the coronary arteries) confirmed the presence of a 95% LAD proximal obstruction. PTCA (balloon angioplasty) and stenting were performed. The patient went home the very next day with his chest feeling "normal." He would be taking Aspirin, metoprolol, Plavix, atorvastatin (to lower cholesterol) and lisinopril (for blood pressure control).

Presently, there are insurance companies who claim that they intend on practicing preventive care but who would probably have rejected Mr. Dear for a stress echo or nuclear study in a doctor's office because the symptoms did not sound "cardiac in origin." Based on my experience, I will say that these companies will argue at length over whether a patient needs to have typical symptoms before they will authorize the above - noted stress tests. A significant number of the doctors working for these insurance companies doing the screening by telephone are not cardiologists. They seem not to know that a routine stress test is only 90% accurate in a man and inexplicably only 66% accurate in a woman. (A stress echo is 95% accurate in both women and men).

These companies will also not cover an ultrafast CT scan of the coronary arteries which will detect calcium and, thus, atherosclerosis that can be followed over the years for progression or regression of the disease.

There are multiple algorithms that exist for how to screen patients with chest pain or who are asymptomatic. The algorithms would have missed Mr. Dear. He could have been sent home and died. At least 80% of patients have as their first symptoms either sudden death or a major heart attack.

There are many people with atypical symptoms such as back pain, jaw pain, elbow pain, pain only in the thumb, and even itching of the nose, which are eventually discovered to be "cardiac," anginal equivalents.

We need better screening plans for atherosclerosis. We also need better blood tests to detect those at risk, including more frequent usage of ultra-fast CT scans of the coronary arteries. These tests detect calcium in the arteries before symptoms or heart attacks occur.

We also need more precise wording, such as:

1. Does your chest feel normal?
2. Do you feel normal?

This may be the difference between interrupting a heart attack and saving a life. Fortunately, Mr. Dear was treated within time and is doing well.

Chapter 37: A Piece of Cake: The Miracle Lady

One of the first patients to come to my practice was an elderly lady on Medicaid who had a heart murmur and was short of breath. She was originally from the Ozarks but she'd moved to Virginia a number of years before. She came to see me and brought her husband in too after she had checked me out. He was over 300 pounds and was in congestive heart failure from weak heart muscle, a cardiomyopathy. He was in worse shape than she was.

Brickie always had a twinkle in her eye and a look of mirth on her face. She gave the impression that she was always sizing up the situation. She loved to tell jokes. She would ask two different couples from her church to give her a ride to her appointment. When both couples showed up, she would simply tell one that she thought their car was more reliable and would be better for going to the appointment. She would tell the other that their car was more comfortable and would be preferable for the leisurely ride home. She would tell both couples that they needed to see me for their blood pressure, high cholesterol, or chest pain. Eventually, both couples became my patients.

Brickie would always call the office before coming in to make sure that we were prepared for her arrival. She liked to have a little piece of cake or a cookie to put her "in the right mood" to see the doctor.

Brickie's husband died of heart failure. Her church was very supportive. She made it through the emotional challenges but she was eventually faced with open heart surgery herself for symptomatic aortic stenosis. Her aortic valve was becoming more and more scarred and narrow, making it hard to breathe and causing chest discomfort and lightheadedness. She needed a new valve.

She decided to push ahead with this surgery which took place smoothly at Fairfax Hospital under the care of its chief of cardiovascular surgery, Dr. Ed Lefrak. The operation was a success but unfortunately Brickie's breast bone was as thin as a pencil. Three days post-op, the wires used to hold her breastbone (sternum) together at the end of surgery eroded through. Brickie contracted a bacterial and fungal infection and was maintained on a respirator for 6 months. I visited almost every day. She always seemed to have that twinkle in her eye and her grip was always strong.

One Sunday, after church, I drove to Fairfax Hospital with two of my small children and visited Brickie in the ICU. The children waved from the hallway. Brickie was still on a respirator but managed an open-eyed smile and a few waves. She later grew stronger and eventually fully recovered and went home. She told me that she knew she was going to make it all along but that seeing my children that day was a real boost. She figured that I wouldn't bring my kids by to see someone who was dying.

Years later, Brickie pressured Dr. Lefrak into having an anniversary celebration to commemorate her indefatigable determination and ability to survive. At the party, Dr. Lefrak presented her a medal which was inscribed with the words: "The miracle lady of Fairfax Hospital." She thanked him for the medal and the kind words but raised her voice to demand: "Now, where's my cake?"

She survived another ten years and was an inspiration to all. She would tell people at church, on the phone, or in the waiting room that if she could survive what she had, then surely they could survive the "measly procedure" they needed. After all, it was just a piece of cake.

Chapter 38: Gunga Din

One day during medical training, I was assigned a new patient from the emergency room. She was a soft-spoken lady of perhaps 35 years of age who had abdominal pain for about a week. There was some nausea but no vomiting or diarrhea. Her pain was somewhat diffuse but more pronounced in the right lower quadrant. She was rather difficult to examine due to extreme overweight - she weighed over 400 pounds, more than the hospital scale could accurately measure. During the examination, my hand and arm up to the elbow would actually completely disappear amidst the abdominal folds as I attempted to palpate organs.

I was quite scrawny back then, still am. At the time, I looked all of 18 years-old. I could have been cast in a movie as the Deputy Sherriff, Don Knotts, in the Andy Griffith show.

Even though the patient denied having a physical relationship for years, I felt it imperative to do a pelvic exam. At the very least, I did not want to be ordering an Upper GI or Barium enema and possibly expose a fetus to radiation.

Back at the Nurses' Station, when I told the nurses my intention, they at first asked if I had lost my mind. There were comments like John McEnroe's infamous: "You can't be serious!" They informed me that there was no exam table that could support the patient. The pelvic exam would have to be done in bed while two nurses held the patient's right leg and another two held the left leg. Their comments just went from there. I was the object of their teasing, not the patient, and it was just their way to establish the pecking order. I was at the bottom. One nurse suggested that they'd tie a rope to my foot just in case they'd lose me.

Returning to the patient, undaunted by their ribbing and equipped with a speculum, I tried a multitude of approaches. Nothing worked. I could not even get a glimpse of the area to be examined much less perform the exam.

I finally gave up. The nurses later said: "We told you so," and "Good job, Johnny Weissmuler!"

Not completely defeated, I nonetheless wrote out the admitting orders. The last thing I wrote for was a urine pregnancy test; while the nurse was reading the orders, I ran for the door. I heard her call out "You are joking, aren't you?"

I returned to the nurse's station the next day and noted their smiles as I asked for the chart. One nurse suggested I might like to check the lab slip taped to the front of the chart. It was the urine pregnancy test. Unbelievable! It *was* positive. As my jaw dropped down to my knees, the nurses chortled: "Well, we guess there's a better man than you somewhere out there, Gunga Din."

The patient was rotated to the appropriate service and I do not know if she eventually delivered her baby safely. But I hope the patient and her baby have since led a healthy and happy life.

Chapter 39: Coming of Age

When I first started practicing Cardiology in 1978, there was only one patient over 90 years of age. She was 106 and still had good mental function and moderate mobility. Unfortunately, she passed away of congestive heart failure within two years.

Her death left me with no patients over 90 for over 20 years. Now I have many more over 90. This is due in large part to modern medicines reducing heart attacks, strokes, and cancers. Less smoking in older patients, dieting, and exercise have played important roles too.

The graphs in the news show the ever-increasing population numbers, the increased percentage of individuals in the over 65-year-old Medicare age group, and it seems there are increasing number of nursing homes and retirement communities. Amazingly, the projections tell us that Medicare is budgeting for lower expenses in the future, not more. How is that possible?

As our aging population increases, we need community health plans and trained personnel to try to help more people stay out of nursing homes and spend their last years safely and comfortably at home when possible. Hospice Programs have been very successful in improving the quality of life towards its end. I hear at a conference that Hospice costs are rising however. We still have to look for efficient, effective models for care for the elderly and debilitated.

Chapter 40: Cruising to a Century

Recently I was paid a visit by a 92-year-old man who has been very active until recently. He'd won gold medals in national track competitions, including the javelin, the shot put, and the discus. He assures me that none of his victories were wind-aided or downhill. Now, he did not feel that he could compete any longer due to a decrease in stamina. He wondered if he should take up a hobby. I suggested that BREATHING become his hobby as it would be a good thing to start to focus on. Breathing deeply periodically throughout the day might help his stamina. Breathing slowly, very slowly, might help him relax, like yoga. I encouraged him to remain positive, that he had survived heart attacks, angioplasty and a pacemaker insertion. He might become the only javelin, shot put, or discus competitor in his age group in 8 years from now when he turns one hundred. Also, he will probably win all three golds just by letting the shot, the discus and the javelin roll out of his hands gently to the ground. I recommended that he not celebrate with high-fives or chest-bumps or dunking the shot over a fence. He should probably procure the aid of a family member to pick up his paraphernalia and the heavy medals. Reenergized by these irreverent comments and with a grin from ear to ear, he promised me a video of the events, already a clear goal and bright vision in his mind.

I hope to learn of his victories.

Chapter 41: LEFTY

Mrs. Williams is a bubbly 92-year-old lady who lost her husband 20 years ago. He used to drag her out bowling and convinced her to join his club. After his death, the members were very supportive and urged her to come out and bowl more frequently. So she did.

What she may have lacked in skill and coordination, she made up for in persistence and determination. Years ago, she was in a heated contest with another lady 20 years younger. The score was tied, 76 to 76, going into the last frame. She took her time and focused on the pin in the center. Then she took 7 long steps and slung the ball past her leg. She sslluuunngg it as hard as she could. Yes, she did. But she forgot to let go of the ball. She did. She forgot. She went flying down the alley a few yards, landing hard on her right arm, and breaking several bones in her hand and wrist. After surgery, she said her arm looked like a 1960's jungle gym, with perpendicular metal bars all over the place.

Never one to be dismayed, Mrs. Williams went back to bowling within a few months. Since her right arm had not healed completely, she decided to go at it with her left. Her progress has been slow but steady over the last few years. She proudly reports that she bowls her age most of the time. A couple of times, she has scored above 100. She brags that this is better than the "kids," the seventy-year olds, with whom she competes.

At the end of a visit she always asks: "Well, how am I doing?" I always answer: "You're doing great, Lefty. Just remember to let go of the ball."

Chapter 42: Sweet Dreams, Sweetheart

A seventy-year old gentleman came to see me again after a three-year absence. We discussed his present and past symptoms. He was examined and recommendations were made, including for a return visit.

On the way out of the room, he asked if I remembered what I had said to him years before when he had first met me. I didn't. He explained that his son was graduating from medical school and was going into anesthesiology. In addition, he was marrying a classmate who was also going into anesthesiology. I remarked that the lucky twosome could get an early start on dotage by taking turns putting each other to sleep at night. He smiled and laughed, as I encouraged him to stay awake and keep his appointments. Suggestions go down better with just a pinch of humor. He kept his appointments from then on.

Chapter 43: Again: Death [Out of Nowhere]

The chart on the door bore the name of a dear lady, a medical colleague, a long-term patient, a person who has always been fun to see. I walked into the examining room with a cheerful smile on my face asking: "How are you? Good to see you." But her sad face and quick response: "Not well, sorry to say," brought an immediate change in my demeanor. She explained that one of her children, a young male adult, was found dead, possibly of a heart attack, at home, alone. The shock, the devastation and the guilt were palpable. She explained how a few days earlier he had felt gassy discomfort in the chest which was relieved by antacids. She had reassured him that it was probably his stomach. "Should I have told him to call 911? Was there any way to know?" I told her that there was no way she could have known then or even now knows what the cause of death was. Even an autopsy may be unable to clarify whether death was due to an arrhythmia, a cardiomyopathy, a stroke, a blood clot to the lung, or a seizure. Experience teaches that feeling guilty is almost universal, especially when death comes suddenly and unexpectedly. Doctors, nurses, parents, siblings, spouses, and friends all feel as though they missed subtle signals or early forewarnings. The overwhelming majority of the time (80%), there are no signs of arteriosclerosis until the heart attack or sudden death occur.

Her son had major challenges which the family had helped him meet. He had a job, a home, a car. He was happy. He did not suffer. She had done a good job. She was an outstanding mother. She must be thankful for the years of memories, both the good ones and the bad ones. She should continue all the wonderful relationships that her son and her family have established and grow new ones. She must continue to spread the caring, the hope and the love with which she surrounded her son (and her patients).

It hurts. It will probably always hurt, maybe a bit less with time. Try to re-channel the pain. Cast off the guilt. You done good, lady. Be proud.

There were tears. There was a good hug. I believe there was a modicum of peace of mind. Thanks were expressed.

Please, let me thank you for sharing all of this and allowing me to be of some small help. I will not forget the privilege that you bestowed upon me. Thank you again.

Chapter 44: A Very Good Laugh

Fairly often an adult child brings an elderly parent to see me, sits patiently through the visit, and occasionally interjects some important symptom or change in status.

One day a sixty-year old daughter brought her eighty-five-year-old father for a follow-up visit after a brief hospitalization for congestive heart failure. He was still experiencing some shortness of breath and edema in spite of two diuretics.

I reiterated what I had advised prior to hospital discharge, which included restriction of sodium, limitation of fluids, and frequent elevation of the legs. As frequently has happened in the past, the gentleman declared that he loved salt, hated pepper and herbs, was tired of having a dry mouth, and intended on drinking anything he wanted.

Before I could open my mouth, the daughter belted out: "So Dad, you either cut back on salt and limit fluids and elevate your legs or...you die!" Both the daughter and her father burst out laughing belly-laughs for almost a minute. I laughed too, longer than they did.

After things settled down, the father agreed to try adhering to the recommendations. His funk had passed.

I reminded him there might be something more objectionable than death that could result from poor choices, namely going back into the hospital, having to eat hospital food, endure a fluid limitation, and lie there with his legs in the air.

Chapter 45: Who Cares for the Dead?

In January, 2015, a Medicare spokesperson said he was pleased to announce to the press that in 2014, Medicare sent out fewer than 50,000 checks for healthcare to dead people. This was exciting, good news for three reasons: First, it was fewer checks Medicare paid for healthcare to dead people than in 2013. Second, it was fewer than the food stamps sent out by the Department of Agriculture to dead people. Third, it was fewer than the welfare checks sent out by the government to dead people.

In June of 2015, an independent investigation estimated that in the 2012 presidential election, there were about 3 million dead people who voted. (An Irish colleague told me that in Ireland the dead voting would be shrugged off with, "At least it was a day out for them.") There is a fair amount of criticism about our country's healthcare system and how we take care of the living. There is general agreement that there is room for improvement. Nevertheless, no one should criticize how we care for our dead. We provide for adequate food (after all they are dead), entertainment money, and healthcare. And we allow them to vote (later than you think) and vote often.

We should not leave out the IRS from the mix. The IRS does not seem to be able to determine who has died. They continue to send dead people tax forms, according to the news.

However, in the meantime, computer hackers are able to hack into the IRS computer system and determine not only who is dead but what their birthdate and social security number is. They then submit an income tax return claiming a refund. I understand it is also the case that hackers can get the names and pin numbers of dead doctors off the Medicare computers and get millions of dollars of false healthcare claims. In addition, hackers can get all the needed data to submit IRS tax forms of anyone alive, file early in January, and obtain the refund. To the casual observer, it would appear that the crooks are smarter than the good guys. How have we left ourselves open to such abuses of technology? Is this not truly regress as opposed to progress?

Chapter 46: Mevacor: Another Breakthrough Medicine

In 1968 during my second year in medical school, Dr. Bill O'Brien conducted a course on preventive medicine. Among other issues he discussed the pharmaceutical companies and the FDA. We were told that Parke-Davis had been fined for promoting a new antibiotic, chloramphenicol, for bronchitis, claiming that it was a kind of "cure-all" with no side effects. It was prescribed widely. Thousands of people developed aplastic anemia. Their bones were unable to make blood cells. It was a fatal condition for most. Doctors' children were affected in great numbers. After the company was punished minimally as some saw it , the company shifted its advertising to other countries. We were shown slides from ads in Italy claiming no side effects. The person in charge of the FDA's investigation and recommendation of a light punishment, we were told, became a vice president at Parke-Davis.

Over 50% of my class chose not to accept gifts from drug companies, including the traditional black bag senior gear. I decided years later not to meet with drug detail people and, as a rule, not to prescribe a new medicine until it had been in general use for one year.

In around 1984 Mevacor (the first statin, lovastatin) was released. I reviewed the studies and was impressed with the data and decided I would prescribe the medicine in order to significantly reduce the risk of heart attack. It was well-established by the Framingham study that for every 1% decrease in the total cholesterol there is a 2% reduction in heart attack, regardless of whether this was accomplished by diet, exercise, high fiber intake (Metamucil or Konsyl), or cholesterol lowering medication. Mevacor was able to surpass all of the above with a reduction of risk by 50% or more.

One day the drug rep for Mevacor peeked through the waiting room door and said he knew I did not as a rule speak to his ilk but could he leave brochures. I told him I would speak to him only on one condition: that he would set up a program for those who could not afford the medication to obtain it for free. He said he would (He Did!). I told him I did not need to speak to him as I had already had reviewed the studies and was going to prescribe Mevacor. Six months later he informed me that I was prescribing more Mevacor than anyone in the DC area. He was getting a promotion into an administrative position. I thanked him for arranging free medication for patients and urged him to continue the program here and expand it wherever he could.

Since then, lovastatin has been replaced by pravastatin, simvastatin(Zocor), atorvastatin(Lipitor), and then rosuvastatin(Crestor). Each one is approximately 20% more effective than its precursor. For some people, liver blood tests go up mildly but do not indicate permanent damage. When the statin is stopped, the tests generally return to normal. There are others, perhaps 1-3%, who may have muscle aching. A blood test for muscle, CPK, may indicate muscle inflammation which in severe cases may cause reduced kidney function. In almost 34 years of prescribing statins, I personally have never seen any patient hospitalized for any negative effect of any medicine for lowering cholesterol.

The fear of problems with many medicines is often exaggerated by the media. The facts reveal that the number one medicine resulting in hospitalization is aspirin. It can cause gastritis, stomach ulcers, bleeding, anemia, passing out, blood transfusions and death. Advil (ibuprofen) is number two for the same reasons. This is rarely reported on the news. The news has morphed into a vehicle of entertainment rather than a source of information or means of education. The news is able to keep us tuned in if the story evokes the following emotions: fear, hatred, anger, jealousy. Possibly 90% of the news is the opposite of uplifting. Bad news sells.

Muscle aching from a statin may be avoided or improved with Co Q10 400 mg qd, magnesium oxide 400 mg qd, or quinine tonic water. Switching from one statin to another may result in improvement in or disappearance of muscle aching.

There are three new medicines approved in 2016 by the FDA. All are injections. All are expensive. No one is rushing to use them and insurance does not generally cover them.

However, what is striking about the data submitted to the FDA is that each medicine may reduce the bad cholesterol, the LDL (Low Density Lipoprotein, L for Lousy) to 25. This may bring about another 25% reduction in the risk of heart attack, stroke, and dementia. Importantly, there are no major side effects yet reported from the medicines. Of equal importance, there is no disease of too low a cholesterol yet.

The number of heart attacks and strokes is decreasing. The statins, with Mevacor's introduction, have played a major role. There will be better medications in the future. These are wonderful contributions. But I think we still need to consider appropriate regulation of pharmaceutical company practices, as we were taught so many years ago.

Chapter 47: Where Goes My Stethoscope?

In the spring of 1969 during my second year of medical school at UVA, we were given a short course in physical examination. One day, one of the professors was teaching us "all about" the stethoscope. He talked for about 25 minutes covering various points including some history, different brands, the function of the diaphragm and bell. He described what to listen to in different places of the body: the arteries, lungs, heart, and intestines.

He then took 20 of us students into a room with a patient who had volunteered for this exposure. He examined the lady and then stepped back and gestured to one of my classmates to step forward and listen to the patient's heart. He stepped forward and began by placing the diaphragm near the left sternal border and then moving to the apex of the heart. It was a good start but not the best one. He had forgotten to put the ear pieces into his ears. I could see that he was somewhat bewildered but could not figure out why he couldn't hear anything. At least 30 seconds passed. I was becoming quite anxious for Peter who was a gentle, soft-spoken, somewhat serious person who would not enjoy being ribbed all around the school if this went on any longer. I stepped to Peter's side and quickly whispered: "Peter, it will probably work better if you put it in your ears," gesturing to the tubes still hanging around his neck. He adjusted his stethoscope, listened a bit, and offered to me: "Much better, thanks."

Years later, around 1992, a colleague was in the office searching for his stethoscope everywhere. He checked all the examining rooms twice, the lunch area, even the front desk.

Finally, he approached me and asked if I had seen it anywhere. I replied that he would do well to check right under his nose. He glanced downward and spotted it on his chest still hanging from his neck. He cracked up. After a few seconds, he asked if I had ever done that. I said I had not but I recounted the story of my classmate and opined that he had surpassed that situation by far. It was hilarious that a well-balanced Board- certified cardiologist could not find a stethoscope hanging from his neck.

Chapter 48: Impersonal Trainer?

An eighty-year old gentleman whom I had cared for over 3 decades came in for a routine office visit. He had undergone successful, life-saving bypass surgery in the 1970's. Ever since then he had been following advice regarding diet, medication, and exercise. He had been walking daily for 30 minutes. Whatever he was doing was working. He was trim, feeling great, and had no symptoms.

The previous week he had been approached by a pleasant young woman who offered to be his "personal trainer." She would outline a program involving not only "cardio" exercise, but also isometric, weight lifting. I explained that isometric exercises did not necessarily extend the lifespan. In fact, it is joked that cardio exercise (walking, jogging, biking, swimming) only increase the lifespan by an average of 3 years. It requires so many hours of exercise that one actually spends more time exercising than there is payback.

Anyway, I said he was in good shape and it was his choice whether or not to keep the trainer. He replied that he needed a note saying it was OK. I asked if I could write that he should continue regular exercise as he had been doing for decades and that he could exercise at home, outside, or at a club. Finally, I asked why the trainer needed a note from me. Was she going to have him do things that are dangerous? He said "No. She obviously just wants to cover her butt!" I asked: "Who's to cover my butt?" It didn't seem that the addition of supervision would be medically necessary. Why should the whole country be held hostage and deemed responsible for activities that are considered normal, advisable and healthy? I offered to give him a copy of his stress test if that would help. I told him he had been doing a great job with his diet, his adherence to medication, and exercise. I urged him to keep it up.

Chapter 49: Patient-Responsibility: Part I

Some studies show that after a heart attack many people stop taking one or more of their medicines. There are 4 medicines that prevent another heart attack: aspirin (40% reduction of risk), a beta-blocker (atenolol, metoprolol, 25% reduction), an ACE inhibitor (lisinopril, 30% reduction), and a statin (atorvastatin, up to 50% reduction). In England, in one study, 90% of patients stopped one medicine by 3 months post heart attack and three medicines by 9 months. There have been proposals to reduce the problem of non-compliance by putting all four pills into one. This may work for those who can swallow large pills but it is an imperfect solution. What doses would be selected?

Human nature is such that patients are reluctant to take their pills, forget, or run out. Sometimes they can't afford the pills.

Multiple approaches are needed. Pill boxes that hold a week's supply help. Phone calls from nurses, relatives, and friends help. Notification by pharmacies of missed refills help. Perhaps financial incentives should be considered. Japanese companies and Safeway are making contracts with employees with annual bonuses for weight loss, exercise, BP control, sugar control, etc. Why not include compliance with medications?

Wouldn't it be nice to have a Surgeon General like Luke Terry (the 1965 start of warnings on cigarettes) with the energy, strength, and persistence to educate us about our responsibility to ourselves as patients?

Chapter 50: Patient Responsibility: Part II

Every study I have seen over the last 46 years has concluded that over 50% of adult hospitalizations are preventable because they result from preventable disease problems.

Strokes for example are considered preventable because without salting our food, blood pressures are for the most part normal. There are thousands of valleys in New Guinea which do not have salt and there are no strokes. We in the US have around 800,000 strokes a year with 200,000 deaths. It is maintained that salt kills 200,000 people a year. Salt was previously used as a preservative. It is no longer needed as such. A German tavern owner centuries ago created the salted pretzel in order to sell more beer. Today, even the cereals have high levels of salt. We are poisoning ourselves with salt.

We are harming ourselves with tobacco products, alcohol, drugs, fatty foods, man-made sugars, high caloric intake, low exercise levels, chemicals, air pollution, etc.

We need someone such as the Surgeon General to focus on programs of prevention. We need employers and educators to focus on health issues.

Perhaps having 11-18-year olds spend time on a Saturday volunteering or simply observing in the emergency rooms could help. They could provide statistics and report what they observed: accidents, drugs, heart attacks, STD's, emphysema, and how that experience affected their choices of healthful living practices.

Chapter 51: Scientific Studies

I often wonder how many studies base their results on assumptions that the patients are taking their medicine and are truthful about missing meds. There was a study published perhaps 5-10 years ago that concluded that perhaps 10% of patients were aspirin resistant since they did not exhibit a reduction in platelet clumping in the blood tests. For a number of years there were reports, conferences, and recommendations on what to do with these folks. Then someone got the bright idea to locate the people identified as aspirin resistant and redo the study, but with one difference. Each person had to come to the study center and take the aspirin under direct observation. The results showed that the number of people who were aspirin resistant was ZERO!

Other studies may be invalid because of too few patients enrolled to demonstrate a statistical benefit. Still other studies are terminated early because early on there is benefit which is fading with time. Researchers need to publish (or perish). They need continuous grants. 80% of published studies show a positive result. Only 20% of studies showing a negative set of findings are published.

Studies need to be scrutinized over a long period of time and verified. The news hardly ever reports on a negative study which fails to support the postulated theory. The news is also slow to retract what has been reported previously but later found to be incorrect.

Consumers cannot do a good job of practicing prevention if they are not given access to correct, up-to-date information.

Chapter 52: Heart Statistics

Statistics regarding heart attacks can be as misleading as those in other areas. There are approximately 1.2 million heart attacks per year (down from a peak years ago of 1.6 million). There are 500,000 deaths (compared to 5,000 with cervical cancer, 20,000 prostate, 30,000 colon, 50,000 breast and over 100,000 lung cancer) per year. Perhaps 40% of the heart attack deaths occur instantaneously without warning. Many occur overnight while asleep. A low percentage occur at work. Circadian rhythms have been implicated. The liver supposedly makes more LDL at night. LDL once oxidized (by iron, homocysteine et al) increases the tension in the "pimple"-like lesion in the wall of the coronary artery that results in bursting and injury to the wall. Platelets (contracted by aspirin, clopidogrel, et al) come to seal off the injury and inadvertently close off the entire artery, causing muscle damage to the oxygen-deprived tissues and abnormal rhythms including sinus arrest (no heart beat).

If one is lucky enough to have a witnessed cardiac arrest with rapid institution of CPR (chest compressions without mouth-to-mouth oxygenation) and defibrillation (if there is a heart rhythm called ventricular fibrillation and not sinus arrest) and one survives to the hospital, then the chance of leaving the hospital with an intact brain can be as good as 15%. Otherwise, unwitnessed arrest has a rate of survival of approximately 5%.

If one has chest pain but does not have an arrest and makes it to the hospital but does not have a blockage of a coronary that can be opened up, the mortality rate is 12-15%.

Balloon angioplasty and stenting can reduce the mortality rate to 4%.

To prevent a second heart attack, one can prescribe aspirin (40% reduction of risk), ACE inhibitor (lowers BP, risk reduction 30%), beta-blocker(limits heart rate, 25% risk reduction), and a statin(lowers LDL, 50% reduction depending on dose, etc.)

For every medicine that is tested and found beneficial, the "relative" reduction is emphasized or reported as opposed to the "absolute" percentage reduction. For example, if an ACE inhibitor such as lisinopril is found in a study to have reduced the mortality rate from 9% to 6%, this is reported as a 33%(3/9) relative risk reduction. However, the actual reduction is 3%, from 9 to 6. This is exaggerating the importance of the data. It may be useful in scientific discussions regarding comparisons of medications but can be confusing to patients who need hard data (absolute numbers) for making important choices.

Chapter 53: How to Spoil a Good Kiss

Cervical cancer is the result of infection with Human Papilloma Virus(HPV). Males are not usually afflicted but are carriers who transmit the germ to females via sexual intercourse. This is one of several sexually transmitted diseases(STD's).

Over 10 years ago, the HPV vaccine was made available but was limited to females between the ages of perhaps 10 to 27. Males were not vaccinated.

Now there are both young women and men who have HPV related throat cancer which is presently difficult to treat, to say the least.

It is apparent that the virus is spread not just by participating in oral sex but also likely from kissing.

For adults, the present recommendation is for up to 27 years of age. It is assumed that people over 27 have already been exposed. Depending on one's situation, one may not have been exposed and may benefit from the vaccine. One should check with one's primary care doctor or gynecologist.

See, NEJM Sept. 29, 2016 page 126g

Chapter 54: Beyond Placebo Effect

In a study on arthritis symptoms, one-third of patients were given Advil labelled as Advil, ⅓ received placebo labelled as Advil and ⅓ were provided placebo labelled as placebo. The results were that benefit was provided to 30% of group 1, 30% of group 2, and 40% of group 3. Placebo labelled as placebo was the best of the lot.

The authors postulate that people are so afraid of prescribed medications that when that fear is eliminated, they believe that only good can come of it. Therefore, they are more relaxed, less worried, less intense and likely to have a higher pain threshold. Homeopathic medicine may work similarly.

At present, it is judged unethical to use a placebo. An example of a placebo treatment that is currently considered inappropriate practice is Vitamin B12 injections in certain circumstances. B12 shots are only allowed if the blood level is low and the patient is not absorbing B12 in the intestine (due to lack of Intrinsic Factor). This is called Pernicious Anemia. It should be noted that Vitamin B12 is available as a pill that can be absorbed under the tongue.

I wonder what the benefit might be from certain sham procedures. In the 1960's, the Vineberg procedure involved opening the chest and implanting the internal mammary artery into the heart muscle, not into the left coronary artery as it is today. Nonetheless, 30% of patients had relief of angina probably due to the placebo effect.

A forty-year old obese man came to me with heart issues. He was unable to give up juices, reduce calories, keep a food log, exercise, attend Weight Watchers, etc. He struggled for months. He finally had a gastric bypass operation. Three months later he was down 30 pounds. He was dieting, keeping a log, exercising, etc. I asked how he had finally come to buy into the diet and exercise programs. He said he was not going to have wasted all that money and discomfort involved in the surgery. He came to the conclusion that the operation alone was not enough. I asked if he thought that a sham procedure would have had the same results. He answered without hesitation: “Probably.”

There are others who have gastric bypass surgery and drink high calorie drinks all day, overcoming the benefits of the operation.

The human mind works mysteriously. One tries to connect, understand, and empathize with patients. The best course may be elusive. One should consider perhaps a support group, hypnosis, homeopathy, anxiety reducing medications or techniques, change of scenery, or other opinions. One must be persistent and supportive.

Further studies on the placebo effect are necessary.

Chapter 55: Placebo Effect, Continued

A recent article in the Washington Post describes genetic studies which indicate that people have different capabilities of achieving a placebo effect. By reducing the number of subjects in a study who have high placebo response, one can conduct more efficient and less costly studies. Also, if someone is highly susceptible to a placebo effect, it would be cheaper to heal their problem with a placebo. However, this would require a change in rules from the Boards of Medicine since prescribing a placebo is considered unethical. Further inquiry in the placebo effect area could bear fruit for patients and the healthcare system.

Chapter 56: The Flu Vaccine: Part One

In 1984, one of my children became sick with the flu the second week of December and stayed home for several days. The third week of December saw a second child kept home from school due to the flu. The third child became ill with the flu during the fourth week of December. And finally, my wife came down with the flu in January. I did not contract the flu during that month-long siege because I had taken the vaccine (a single valent dose of the previous year's mutant offspring). Neither my wife nor our children had received the vaccine. After that I made sure the children received the vaccine in September and they did not catch the flu after that.

The Flu Vaccine: Part Two

When my youngest son was a senior in high school, he greeted me upon my arrival home from work one day with the following declaration: "Dad, I hate you." I replied: "Yes, I know. This is not the first time you have expressed your antithetical love with such bravado. But, pray tell, what now prompts this joyous salutation?" He grieved: "Do you know how many of my classmates were in school today?" I guessed: "Twenty?" He formed a circle with his thumb and index finger and raised his hand next to his mouth and iterated "None!" He then questioned: "Do you know how many of my teachers were in school today?" I smiled inquisitively: "Three?" He raised his hand circled like an O and re-iterated: "None!" The cross-examination continued: "Do you know what I did all day at school?" I inquired: "Did you wash blackboards?" I thought this might throw him off track as he might not know what a blackboard was. It didn't work. "Dad. This is serious. I spent the whole entire day alone in a study hall with nothing to do since there were no teachers handing out assignments. Next year, I am not getting the vaccine. I would rather stay home like all the other miserable people, watching television and eating bon bons." I replied, "OK, but did you not consider fleeing your abandoned school for home since there was no one to stop you? I suggest you keep that in mind for next year." "Thanks Dad, I hate you."

The Flu Vaccine: Part Three

My wife's maternal grandfather came to New York City from Rome, NY, having skipped college. He sailed through Columbia P&S (medical school), then turned down a post medical school fellowship in Europe to marry and start a family. He opened an office in his home on 46th street and Eighth close to NYC's theatre district. He recounted his memory of when the flu pandemic hit Manhattan in 1918 to my wife in a letter. He would leave his home/office in the morning to see his patient(s) and start working his way up the stairs of one brownstone building, cross the roof to another, and work his way down the neighboring building, trying to see the sick and dying who wanted his help. There was little he could do. He wrote of their misery. All he had to offer was aspirin, fluids, comfort and hope. He was known to give money to those who could not afford medicine.

Decades later when the flu vaccine was made available, he was overjoyed. He told me he hoped that no one would have to relive the horror of the pandemic that took thousands of lives. (Amazingly, neither he, his wife, nor any of their many children came down with the flu.)

The Flu Vaccine: Part Four

My wife, like many others, was leery of the flu vaccine for a number of years. Now she not only gets the vaccine, but she has become an advocate. I was amazed by how much she absorbed during my last two years of medical school and my subsequent medical training. I can come home and hear her on the phone advising someone about a medical condition. It is amazing how she can question various sorts of advice given her but later hand out the same advice to others. After she hangs up, I usually pounce from the other room, asking: "How do you spell the word hypocrite?" I then spell her name in response. Secondly, I wonder out loud if I am obligated to report her for practicing without a license.

Her grandfather would be proud. Poppa always thought Jeanne's mother should have become a physician.

The Flu Vaccine: Part Five

The flu vaccine used to contain a single species of virus, either influenza A or influenza B. Now it may contain 3 or 4 species in one vaccine. It has to be more effective now.

The flu virus mutates every year. One can never have the same virus in the vaccine that is actually infecting people today.

Receiving the vaccine exposes you to a weakened form which is highly unlikely to kill you. It is like exposing you to a chihuahua so you are fortified and better able to fight a Great Dane when it attacks. It is like sending you a picture or a profile of a criminal so that your immune system recognizes and responds more quickly.

The vaccine does not prevent you from breathing in the virus or getting infected. It tips the balance in your favor so that hopefully you won't die. We were taught in medical school that the way to assess the efficacy of the flu vaccine was to count the number of deaths from pneumonia that year. The flu virus generally weakens the immune system so that it cannot fend off the Streptococci bacteria. There are usually 10,000 deaths a year from pneumonia.

On Labor Day weekend, perhaps it was in 2013, the University of Maryland and American University quarantined their students because of so many cases of the flu. The virus mutates each year in chickens in Asia and is brought to the west coast and then the east coast by returning students and tourists. No one can really predict when it will hit or when it will peak. I take it and prescribe it starting before Labor Day. It takes 2-3 weeks to reach full protection. I have yet to see someone sick in March who took the vaccine in September.

The British have data on most of their citizens which indicate that those receiving the flu vaccine have fewer heart attacks than those who don't. Perhaps fortifying the immune system does help reduce heart attacks. If so, what about strokes?

The Flu Vaccine: Part Six

One fall, a husband and wife made different choices. She received the flu vaccine. He didn't. In January, he came to the ER with severe shortness of breath, fever, weakness, and a productive cough. His blood tests later confirmed he had the flu. His sputum revealed staphylococcus aureus, a very unkind, virulent bacterium. He ended up on a respirator with paralysis for over 3 months. Luckily, he survived.

His wife also had a fever and a cough. A gram strain of the sputum (phlegm) was consistent with Staphylococcus. This was later confirmed by culture. She was begun on antibiotic pills and went home from the ER. She was barely symptomatic in spite of being infected.

The Flu Vaccine: Part Seven

Every year there is a statement on the news by a government representative that there will be no shortage of flu vaccine this year, there will be 80 or 90 million doses available, so everyone in the country can get one. Since there are 300 million people in the country, this must be inaccurate. The newscasters have yet to ask how this makes sense.

Chapter 57: Mother-in-Law vs. Death

My mother-in-law was born in New York City, at home, on 46th street, in 1912. She graduated from college at age 19, taught French, and raised 4 children.

In her later years, she would read several books a month. She would pass along which books she felt were worth reading. We would at our next visit discuss the contents of the books. Her taste in reading material was top notch and my wife and I looked forward to her next recommendations; we thought of her as our book club. She remained mentally sharp until her last months.

Over the years, she had survived a number of malignant cancers. In her last several years, she suffered from arthritis and was unable to get up and around without assistance.

Nevertheless, she maintained her sense of humor until the end. At some time in the recent past, she was washing the dishes with one of her granddaughters-in-law when the latter asked her if she got the same relaxing, comforting feeling that she did from having her hands in the sink in warm water. My mother-in-law looked closely at her granddaughter-in-law and with astonishment queried: “Are you well?”

When she was 99 years old, we were alone when she said: “You know, Bill, I am now praying for death. I have lived long enough.” I replied with a grin that “It has taken 50 years, but we are now praying for the same thing.” She smiled broadly and said: “Touché. That was a good one.” She died in 2016 at age 103.5 and I am sure she was fast- tracked to heaven. Moreover, Gabriel.

Chapter 58: Mother-in-Law: A Digression

When my mother-in-law was between 66 to 80 years old, after Jeanne's father passed away, she would occasionally come to visit. She would generally stay a week (an entire week!). During that week, she would spend 2 full days matching socks that had been separated or lost a mate somewhere between the bedrooms, the washing machine and the dryer. There were two large plastic baskets full of unmatched socks. She would reunite about 50 pairs and set aside another 25 unmatched pairs. I, of course, was especially grateful for the money that we saved from buying fewer socks.

On the other hand, I was always hoping she might finish this tortoise-like activity more expeditiously and then tackle some other much-neglected tasks (she admired my rubber band and string collections), and be able to leave maybe two or three days earlier – to her and my relief.

I racked my brain trying to come up with a solution. Perhaps the sock manufacturers could place a velcro square on each sock. No, they profit from lost socks. That's why they have not come up with a solution for this age-old, world-wide problem.

I noticed while checking the legs of patients for edema that many men were wearing unmatched socks. I would chuckle at this flawed dress code and joke: "I bet you have another pair just like it at home."

Then it finally hit me. All one has to do is place a safety-pin on one of the socks. When taking off the other sock, immediately pin it to its mate. Leave the safety-pin in place for the life of the sock. It was a miracle. My mother-in-law was skeptical at first but then she had to admit the system worked. She saw that her services were less necessary. She reduced her stays to five days at a time and joy returned to Mudville (i.e., her and me) a little sooner.

Chapter 59: STATISTICS Can Lie

In 1970 or so, there was a study about phlebitis (blood clots in the legs) in women. The study compared 1,000 women taking BCP (Birth Control Pills) with 1,000 not taking BCP. The study period was 1 year. The results revealed that there were 3 women on BCP with phlebitis versus 1 case in the Non BCP group. This is a difference of 2 people per 1,000 or .2%. This is not scary in the least. However, the authors concluded and the headline in the news stated that there was a 300% increase in phlebitis on "the pill." This is clearly a distortion of the facts in order to gain recognition and more research money. Bad news sells!

And on that note....The media thrive on 4 emotions: fear, anger, hatred, and jealousy. Consider the weather, for example. The weather report used to be no more than 2-3 minutes long. Now it's at least 5 minutes and sometimes 30 minutes or all day. Your attention is grabbed by something bad happening, likely not in your area, but which might reach your area or affect distant relatives or friends. Newscasters seem to get new outfits they can model while "on the scene" such as a hurricane.

The sports report on the news no longer showcases a preponderance of athletic prowess but focuses on contracts, money, harassment, fights, disagreements, trades and games to be played that night or the next day. In fact, both the weather person and the sports person consistently tell the viewer when the weather is OK to get out to the park early and support the home team. Upcoming events seems of more interest than discussion of what it occurred in recent athletic contests. It is a different kind of journalism.

Chapter 60: All Balled uP

A cardiology colleague signed out to me on a Friday afternoon a patient with an enlarged scrotum. It was huge - bigger than a grapefruit. It was! He was admitted to the hospital and a urologist was asked to see him the next morning to diagnose the problem and recommend appropriate treatment. The working diagnosis was a hydrocele, a collection of fluid due to a narrowing of the spermatic cord.

The next morning I happened upon the urologist walking down the hallway and I inquired whether or not he had seen the patient yet. He said: "I did." I asked what the problem was. He responded in a low voice, briefly: "Congestive heart failure. I'd suggest Lasix" (a diuretic).

I thanked him as he turned on his heels and headed for the door. I found the patient, examined him, and noted the absence of neck vein distention, rales in the chest (a sign of fluid), an S3 heart gallop, enlarged liver, or leg edema.

I respectfully noted the 2-sentence consultation from the urologist (who was decades older than me) and dutifully ordered the Lasix diuretic.

The next morning, Sunday, the man felt much better. He had lost 5 pounds and his scrotum was normal. He went home.

On Monday, I told my cardiology colleague that over the weekend I had the most fascinating case of congestive heart failure with no neck vein enlargement, rales, S3, enlarged liver, or edema. He asked how I was able to make the diagnosis. I said: "I wasn't. The urologist did. It was your patient with the enlarged scrotum." He chuckled. So much for the textbooks. So much for present day 4 page consultations.

Chapter 61: Jogging?

One day several years ago, a seventy-year old patient who had survived coronary bypass surgery and angioplasty came to the office for a treadmill stress test. He was about five feet nine and weighed in at 250 pounds. He kept a towel around his neck, which had a pinkish hue to it(the neck, not the towel). He was bothered by a shortness of breath with a minimum of exertion. His exercise on the treadmill was limited but there were no signs of strain on the EKG.

After the test was completed and he had recovered his breathing, he told me that he had been "jogging" recently outside in his neighborhood. He was chugging along at a steady pace without either foot actually leaving the ground. At some point, a pink Cadillac pulled up and stopped next to him. There was a young boy sitting in the passenger seat on the right side of the car. An elderly lady leaned over from the driver's seat and inquired: "Excuse me sir, can you help us?" The patient replied: "Certainly ma'am. How can I be of service?" "Well," she said, "My grandson's turtle escaped from his enclosure and we wondered if he might have passed you going in this direction." He said he had not spotted the escapee but he would certainly keep an eye out. With a big grin, the lady thanked him profusely, stepped on the gas, and roared off. The man resumed his "jogging", scanning the horizon for wayward turtles. A jog is not necessarily a jog.

Chapter 62: Alzheimer's Disease and Statins

The label of Alzheimer's Disease(AD) is given to those patients with cognitive deterioration (memory loss) who do not have evidence of a stroke(CVA) on a MRI brain scan. The patients who have evidence of a CVA and dementia are labelled multi-infarct dementia(MID) even if the only evidence of a stroke is one pinhead defect on an MRI. Much attention is focused on the greater buildup of proteins such as amyloid and tau in the brains of those with AD. Very little mention is made of the consistent finding of small vessel disease (a euphemism for arteriosclerosis) on every MRI scan of patients with AD.

Multiple areas of study have shown that steps that reduce arteriosclerosis/atherosclerosis not only reduce heart attack and stroke(CVA) but also reduce Alzheimer's. Reduction of risk may be 50% with six portions of fish per week, 30% with 30 minutes of brisk walking six times per week, 30% with significant weight reduction, 30% with significant blood pressure reduction, 20% with maintaining a normal blood glucose(sugar) of 99 or less, and 25 to 50% with reduction of LDL cholesterol.

Finally, there is a study cited in the Washington Post on December 20, 2016 which concludes that cholesterol-lowering statins reduce Alzheimer's significantly. There is no mention of dosage in the Post but recent studies submitted to the FDA regarding three new injectable medicines for cholesterol indicate that lower is better in regard to LDL levels. There were no specific side effects and no disease attributed to too low a cholesterol.

Recent studies indicate that the population of elderly people is increasing and so is the number of people with AD. However, the percentage of people with AD is decreasing. The authors of the study postulate that cholesterol-lowering medications are responsible. This is likely true, but as noted above, there are multiple steps that patients can take(eating more fish, exercising six times a week, losing weight, lowering BPif elevated, avoiding or reversing high sugar levels) that not only reduce the risk of heart attack(M1) and stroke but also reduce Alzheimer's and multi-infarct dementia.

Chapter 63: Iron: The Number One Oxidant

It is not unusual to hear about the anti-oxidants such as Vitamin C, Vitamin E, B12, B6, and folic acid. However, it is a rarity to hear about the substances they are meant to counteract, the oxidants. Oxidants bring about the oxidation or chemical transformation of LDL(the bad cholesterol) to a form that can build up in the walls of arteries. Iron is the number one oxidant present in the body. The process of rust formation is oxidation.

The evidence pointing to iron as a major culprit in the disease arteriosclerosis(atherosclerosis) is as follows:

1. The rate of heart attacks in women after menopause around age 55, increases suddenly and dramatically. Hormone levels change gradually over a number of years. What changes suddenly is cessation of menses and increased iron levels! [1]
2. The rate of heart attack increases significantly after a hysterectomy without removal of the ovaries in women from age 30 to 55. Hormone levels are unchanged. Menses ceases. Iron levels build up. [2]
3. Hemochromatosis is an inherited disease with increased iron deposition in almost all tissues of the body. There is a higher rate of heart attack in people with the full blown disease and also in those who are carriers (heterozygotes, not a full blown case of the disease). Blood removal, phlebotomy, once per month prevents heart attacks. [3]
4. A protein carrier of iron, ferritin, is elevated(>200 mcg.) in patients with heart attacks. However, since this

protein can also be elevated when an inflammatory reaction occurs, some discount the importance of this finding. However, I have tested scores of patients 3 months after a heart attack and the ferritin is unchanged. [4]

5. Patients undergoing coronary artery bypass surgery who receive a blood transfusion have a higher 2-year mortality rate than those not receiving a transfusion.
6. Hemodialysis patients have a 50% rate of death from heart attack. Because all patients with renal failure are anemic(in large part because of decreased production of erythropoietin), they receive intravenous iron weekly. They also usually receive erythropoietin(Procrit). An ultrafast CT scan of the heart identifies the 50% with arteriosclerosis.
7. Studies comparing blood donors to non-blood donors indicate a decreased risk of heart attack up to 85%. [5,6,7]
8. “Hard” water has higher levels of iron. In counties with “hard” water, the rate of heart attack is higher than in any other counties. In a Scientific American article in the 1970’s, the number of wells in Pennsylvania correlated with the number of heart attacks per county.
9. Studies involving surgery on the chest or in the abdomen reveal that patients who receive a blood transfusion have significantly increased rates of heart attack.
10. Studies of diabetics reveal that high iron levels correlate with higher rates of heart attack.

With all this evidence against iron, one might wonder why the experts have not arrived at a guilty verdict. The reason is that the evidence is circumstantial. A double-blind, controlled, prospective study is needed before a consensus can be reached in the scientific community.

In the meantime, it is reasonable and safe to take the following steps:

1. Donate blood at least 3 times per year. Remember the needs of the country and especially our men and women in the military. Consider donating around Memorial Day, July 4, and Veterans Day. Call the Red Cross at 1-800-GIVE-LIFE and schedule your donation.
2. Avoid iron-rich foods and vitamins fortified with iron. Even many cereals have iron added to them.
3. Avoid "hard" water, well water.

Literature Cited

1. Magnusson, Magnus, et al. Iron metabolism and coronary heart disease. Primary Card. 1995; 21(12):17-20.
2. Sullivan, J.L. The iron paradigm of ischemic heart disease. Am. Heart J. 1989; 117:1177-1188.
3. Sullivan, J.L. Heterozygotes hemochromatosis as a risk factor for premature MI. Med. Hypotheses. 1990 Jan; 31(1): 1-5.
4. Moroy, C., et al. Elevated serum ferritin level in acute MI. Biomed Pharmacother 1997; 51(3): 126-130.

5. Tuomainen, T., et al. Cohort study of relation between donating blood and risk of MI in 2,682 men in eastern finland. Brit. Med. J. March 1997; 314;: 793-794.
6. Salonen, J.T., et al. Donation of blood is associated with reduced risk of MI. Am. J. Eped. Sept. 1998; 148(5): 445-451.
7. Meyers, D.G., et al. Possible association of a reduction in cardiovascular events with blood donation. Heart Aug. 1997; 78(2): 188-193.
8. Knudtson, Merril., et al. Chelation therapy for ischemic heart disease. JAMA. Jan. 23, 2002; 287(4), 481-485.
9. Hu, Frank. Iron Heart Hypothesis. JAMA. Feb. 14, 2007; 297(6), 639-641.

8/6/10

Dysthinkia

Dysthinkia is an unthreatening word,
One which you probably have never, ever heard.
You won't find it listed in the dictionary.
Nor in Dortland's if you should choose to tarry.

It is simply a substitute for other words or phrases,
That usually provoke anger or defensive gazes.
"Non-discerning", "irrational", "ignorant", and "dumb."
For the most part simply don't get the job done.

Dysthinkia describes that state of mind
When a Nobel-Prize winner has suddenly gone "blind."
It may be the glasses atop his head,
By the time he's rebooted he may just be dead.

He could have turned left out of the far right-hand lane,
Causing someone significant life-altering pain.
We all have disconnects in our own little brains,
Which create or contribute to life's daily strains.

Someone may tell us what it is we can't see,
But the brain remains locked with no available key.
Admitting we all have a dysthinkia of sorts,
Is kind of like showing that you too have warts.
A person will listen from a level vantage point,
And is much less likely to get his nose out of joint.

Chapter 64: Memory

Memento is the most thought-provoking movie I have ever seen.

It portrays a young man who suffers from amnesia, which starts shortly after his wife dies of an excessive dose of insulin for her diabetes.

The story is told in a rapid sequence of scenes which could be flashbacks, dreams, imaginings, remembrances, or reality. It is totally confusing until the last five minutes when there is a grand denouement.

It becomes apparent, though it is not stated as such, that the brain has demonstrated a capacity for independent thinking and altering of the facts. This helps to explain why eyewitness testimony is not very reliable and how both parties cannot remember the precise details of an argument.

Self-defensive thought processes may result in incorrect thinking which may impede one's ability to function healthfully and effectively. Whatever the challenge, one must consider verifying the presumed facts and then recording them in a timely fashion. The more time passes, the less accurate one's memory may be.

Chapter 65: Brain on Fire

Brain on Fire by Susannah Cahalan was published in 2013. She tells her story in fluid detail. She was in her twenties when she became acutely ill with fever, malaise, and abnormal thinking. She was hospitalized at NYU in New York and was diagnosed as having schizophrenia of unknown cause. She had a minor elevation of spinal fluid white blood cells. Eventually, she underwent a brain biopsy which revealed a vasculitis. She was treated for this inflammation and recovered over a six-month period. She came very close to being transferred to an institution for the mentally ill, literally a potential dead end.

The story is gripping. One wonders how often a mental illness may actually be due to an undiagnosed physical ailment such as a vasculitis. This book should be recommended reading for Neurologists and Psychiatrists.

Chapter 66: Health Savings Accounts

Two Days that Ruined Your Health Care is a book by William C. Waters III, published in 2008 by Logikon Press Newman, Georgia.

Dr. Waters tells about the passage of the Stabilization Act of 1942 passed on October 2, 1942. The bill allowed employers to deduct from taxable income all payments for employees' health premiums. The employees did not receive the same benefit. Hence, employees forfeited their right to choose whatever health plan they would like. Would anyone give up the right to pick the car of their choice?

On April 10, 1965 President Johnson signed into law the bill establishing Medicare for people over 65 years old. This let the government in the door to pass regulations and eventually set price controls called the DRG system introduced during the Reagan administration.

Dr. Waters argues that insurance itself is the problem because it gives people the impression that someone else is responsible. Government funds pay for 46% of costs. We pay as a country 13% for out of pocket expenses.

Dr. Waters proposes Health Savings Accounts as a potential solution to the problem. First, one obtains a high-deductible insurance(catastrophic policy) to cover major medical problems. Then one sets aside an annual fund pre-tax for ongoing medical expenses. One may use credit or debit cards. If you don't spend the entire amount, it is rolled over to the next year. Excess money left in the fund at retirement can go into an IRA. Not only will this result in a financial savings but it will give back to the consumer control of his insurance.

However this possible solution is not available at present for persons who barely earn enough money to cover their other basic bills like food, shelter and clothing.

Chapter 67: National Health Care in England

After World War II, the British established a National Health Care system with free care for all. During the summer of 1966, I was in London as a volunteer social worker or aide. There was a whole group of us who volunteered under the name of the Winant and Clayton Volunteers. (Gil Winant was our ambassador to England during WWII. His work, support and sensitivity to their plight earned him enormous admiration by the British. Father Clayton was an English minister.)

Midway through my stay I became pretty sick with a sore throat and a high fever. After two days, I was taken to a doctor's office. The waiting room was full of people who were sitting in wooden straight-back chairs. I waited my turn for 90 minutes or so. I was brought into the doctor's office and was seated in a chair in front of his desk. There was no examining table. He asked what the problem was. I indicated I had a sore throat. He stood up and leaned over the desk asking me to say "ahh." He asked if I was allergic to penicillin. He wrote a prescription. He did not take my temperature, nor listen to my lungs or heart. We were done in about 1-2 minutes. I recovered.

I asked numbers of people how the system was. They were all very pleased, because there was no bill.

There is a wonderful book by Henry Marsh called *Do No Harm* that describes the British system and the doctor's experiences. He is a Neurosurgeon who has to struggle with long delays in scheduling a bed and an operation. No one can be admitted or operated on until a bed is actually empty. Nothing can be scheduled after mid- afternoon because the support staff goes off duty at a time certain. If you don't want to wait 3 months for surgery, you can go out of the system, as long as you can pay. The same is true throughout Europe.

My visit with the British doctor now seems very similar to my medical mission trips to Honduras during which I would see 200-300 patients per day. It's overwhelming to stay focused at that level. It is sad, to say the least, to turn people away at the end of the day.

It is true that we have a maldistribution of doctors in this country but I believe we are still better off than most.

Because of the reductions in remuneration for primary care doctors in this country however, only about 1% of medical school graduates are entering primary care. This problem might be helped if federal, state, or local governments contracted with medical students to commit to primary care in a specific town or area in return for reduced or free tuition. Numbers of towns in Maine have gone this route. The alternative may be producing more nurse practitioners to serve in rural or poor areas in primary care positions. When I was a volunteer in the Public Health Service from 1973 to 1975 in Shiprock, New Mexico, I ran a program that educated Navajo high school graduates who were being trained to be Community Health Medics. Jenny Manuelito, Mae Jean Joey, and Chris Chavez passed the tests with flying colors and demonstrated competence out in the community and in the hospital.

Chapter 68: CPR

Cardiopulmonary Resuscitation(CPR) is the name given to the activity undertaken to revive someone who has passed out from a possible heart attack or an abnormal heart rhythm. In addition to chest compressions, it was felt for a long time that mouth to mouth introduction of oxygenated air was critical. Thanks to the careful studies of Dr. Gordon Ewy at the University of Arizona, it is now believed that mouth to mouth is generally counterproductive because it increases pressure in the chest and retards blood flow to the chest and brain.

For years, CPR has produced poor results. Usually, approximately 5% of people receiving CPR have left the hospital 30 days later with an intact brain. This is a result of poor blood flow to the brain for 3 minutes or more. If blood flow is not restored quickly, then one may be able to restart the heart but the brain is already permanently damaged. In Seattle, CPR has been taught in high schools, among other places, with the result being a high proportion of the citizenry are able to institute CPR quickly. The results have been that upwards of 25% of people receiving CPR survived to 30 days.

It is also critical to have a defibrillator available quickly. If the heart rhythm is ventricular fibrillation, then a jolt from a defibrillator can restore the heart rhythm to normal. The airplanes now have automatic defibrillators as do many businesses.

Over 10 years ago, I approached the manager of my local bank and explained the benefits of an Autometer External Defibrillator(AED). He presented the idea to the bank president who turned him down. The manager died of a heart attack at work within six months. Besides the fact that this gentle soul is no longer around, there is also the financial loss involved in finding and training a replacement. Simply put, the decision was a bad business decision.

I have urged family members of those with coronary atherosclerosis or an abnormal rhythm to learn CPR. The Red Cross and local hospitals have convenient and effective courses. The more people who learn CPR, the more people will survive a heart attack. "Witnessed" cardiac arrests with prompt institution of CPR demonstrate far superior results than unwitnessed.

Chapter 69: Dogs and Other Pets

For years, studies have shown that people who have lost a loved one survive longer and have a better quality of life if they have a pet. For some a parakeet works. Others may find comfort with a cat.

A few years ago, there was a story of a family that owned a large pig that stayed in the home. One night a fire started in the basement. The pig detected the smoke and climbed upstairs to the second floor where the family was sleeping. The pig hurled itself against the doors, awakened the family, and led them downstairs. They escaped the fire with their lives, thanks to the pig.

Soon thereafter (Yes, I digress, again), there was a report of a lady who was being carjacked and robbed. She told the thief that she had no cash with her but she had $500 at home, a few blocks away. The thief directed her to drive home, get out of the car, and open the front door. As soon as the door opened, her 200-pound pig launched itself at the thief, knocking him down on the pavement, causing him to lose consciousness. The pig stayed on top of the man until the police arrived.

Dogs are the ultimate service pets. They can detect seizures minutes before they occur and warn their owner so that the person may lie down in a safe place. They also can sense anxiety and stress and can lick the owner's hand or lay their head in his/her lap.

There is a border collie in Budapest who has learned the names of 300 objects which she can bring on command to her owner.

One of the many wonderful dog books I have read is Until Tuesday. The author was a survivor of the war in Iraq. Besides having to deal with an amputation, he suffered from Post-Traumatic Stress Disorder (PTSD). He was chronically depressed and unable to function until he was given a service dog named Tuesday. Tuesday helped him to relax and also helped him navigate when he felt weak or lost his balance. Tuesday gave him confidence and hope for years. The story is well worth reading.

Unfortunately, the news reported that Tuesday's owner died in 2016. He'd dropped Tuesday off to stay with a friend or acquaintance shortly before he died.

I think Tuesday was trained in a program at Dobbs Ferry, NY. We could use a lot more service dogs in many areas and donations are needed to support their upbringing and training.

Chapter 70: Takotsubo's Syndrome; Broken Heart

A mysterious ailment of the heart became apparent about ten years ago. I had neither seen a case nor heard about it until then. It is characterized by symptoms and findings consistent with a heart attack but with normal coronary arteries and usually a complete recovery in a month. The left ventricle (pumping chamber) shows complete inactivity(akinesias) of the heart muscle at the apex (tip of the heart.) The base of the heart is generally hypercontractile(overactive). The resulting silhouette of the heart looks like a lobster pot, which is called Takotsubo in Japanese.

It was first described in Japan. It affects women more than men. It may occur more in people who have lost a loved one. Hence, it has been dubbed the Broken Heart Syndrome.

A news report postulated that the eighty-four-year-old Debbie Reynolds may have experienced Takotsubo's Syndrome one day after the death (by heart attack) of her sixty-year old daughter, Carrie Fisher.* Perhaps excess adrenaline or dopamine plays a role.

*The Washington Post recently reported autopsy results for Carrie Fisher. Without concluding any different cause of death, the report nonetheless evidenced Ms. Fisher's continuing struggle with substances and emotional stability. Debbie Reynolds had much to grieve as a mother.

Chapter 71: Do You Hear What I Hear?

After two years of service as an internist on the Navajo Reservation, I returned in 1975 to complete my last year of residency in Ann Arbor. One of my first rotations was a month-long stint as the resident in charge of the Coronary Care Unit(CCU).

A thirty-eight-year-old woman came to the ER one night with new onset, severe, sharp left chest pain with no radiation of pain, palpitations, shortness of breath, or edema. Her EKG was normal. Her chest pain was atypical and did not fit the pattern of angina or a heart attack. Neither did it exclude the possibility of a heart attack. I examined her briefly and then whisked her off to the CCU because the policy then was to minimize the possibility of dying from Ventricular Tachycardia(VT). Waiting for hours in the ER for the results of blood tests was considered bad form.

After the patient was tucked into bed and hooked up to the monitor leads, I obtained a complete history and performed the customary physical exam. On listening to her heart with my stethoscope, I noted the usual first and second heart sounds with the normal splitting of S2, the absence of a gallop, and the absence of a murmur. However, there was a third heart sound that I had never heard before then.

The next morning on rounds I presented the case to a room full of students, interns and residents and an inquisitive attending(full-time) physician whom I will name Dr. Smart. Dr. Smart grilled me as if I was on the witness stand: "So, you heard an extra sound that you have never heard before?" "Yes," I replied. "Are you sure it's not a gallop?" "Very sure," I answered. "Is it an ejection click as with aortic stenosis or an opening snap of mitral stenosis?" "No. It's in the middle of systole (when the heart is contracting)."

Dr. Smart finally arose from his seat and led the whole troop into the patient's room. He introduced himself and proceeded to listen to the patient's heart. After perhaps 2 minutes, he stood upright and asked me again: "You have never heard this before? Have you ever heard of Dr. Barlow?" "No," I repeated.

Dr. Smart then led us back to the conference room and proceeded to give us a lecture on Barlow's Syndrome, a condition discovered by Dr. John Barlow in South Africa in about 1969. The other name for it is Mitral Valve Prolapse(MVP). The extra sound was called a click and occurs when the mitral leaflet snaps back toward the left atrium when the ventricle contracts. There is often a murmur associated with the click which represents some degree of mitral regurgitation.

In any event, the chest pain was related to the MVP and not a forewarning of a heart attack(MI). The patient was informed of her condition. Propranolol, the only beta-blocker available then, was prescribed and she was discharged.

Dr. Smart advised everyone to lookup MVP in the journals. More importantly, he urged all to listen to the patient's click because it was so easy to hear as long as you were listening for it.

MVP is an inherited condition which is presumably present at birth but infrequently diagnosed until later in life. It exists in perhaps 15% of the population. It is an autosomal dominant characteristic which means that it occurs when only one parent has the trait and has a 50/50 chance of occurring with each child, similar to brown eyes when one parent has brown eyes. Similarly, each sibling has a 50% chance of having MVP.

The diagnosis of MVP is best made by hearing a click with a stethoscope. A mitral late systolic murmur is also proof of MVP being present. An echocardiogram may demonstrate MVP 70% of the time. Not every physician is trained to hear the click or the murmur. Stethoscopes vary in their quality. The best place to listen with a stethoscope is at the left side of the sternum (the breast bone) near to the fifth rib. The best position is with the patient standing, especially after doing 4 knee bends. The faster the heart beats, the better heard is the click and the murmur. Hence, if the patient is relaxed and the heart rate is slow, the diagnostic sounds may not be heard.

MVP may be associated with sharp chest pains, palpitations (extra heart beats or paroxysmal atrial tachycardia), shortness of breath, dizziness, anxiety, panic attacks, migraine headaches, depression, headaches with forehead pain often attributed to sinus problems, fatigue, decreased energy and difficulty sleeping may be present. It is postulated that people with MVP are more sensitive to adrenalin.

Associated physical findings include a high-arched palate (roof of the mouth), pectus excavatum (dipping down of breast bone), pectus carinatum (curving up of the breast bone), kyphosis, or scoliosis.

An EKG may demonstrate a short PR interval (.12 msec or less), PAT, or an RSR in V1. The symptoms of MVP most often respond to a beta-blocker such as atenolol or metoprolol if the heart rate(pulse) is above 60 beats per minute(BPM). The goal of treatment is a resting heart rate of approximately 60 BPM. Beta-blockers counteract some effects of adrenalin. In some people, vigorous exercise (brisk walking 30 minutes, 6 days a week) may have the same effect as medication. In others, the heart rate is already 60 BPM or less and different beta-blockers such as pindolol and sectral are preferable.

People with glaucoma may be treated with eye drops called timolol, a beta-blocker. They may be receiving treatment without knowing it.

Occasionally, a person with MVP may develop severe mitral regurgitation and may require a valve repair or replacement. This is infrequent.

Dr. Proctor Harvey was the Chief of Cardiology at Georgetown University Hospital when I was a fellow. He taught the proper use of the stethoscope, an art which is dying. By example he also taught respect, kindness, and compassion. He always used to say that listening to the heart is like going to the symphony. You may not hear the oboe unless someone alerts you to its presence.

Chapter 72: Can You Please Wash Your Mouth

There is a sneaky germ called Streptococcus viridans which lives in almost everyone's mouth. It does not cause Strep throat or pneumonia. However, if it enters the bloodstream, as it can when the dentist rubs on or nicks the gums, then it can go to the mitral valve that is not normal because of MVP or rheumatic fever et al. The germ can infect the valve and severely injure it. This requires at least 4 weeks of intravenous antibiotics and possibly a new valve. Fortunately, this is infrequent, perhaps 1 person out of five-thousand dental visits.

For fifty years, penicillin pills were recommended for prevention of a heart valve infection, "subacute bacterial endocarditis" (SBE). It seemed to work very well.

Ten years ago, a Heart Association Committee recommended switching from penicillin to amoxicillin since the latter was perhaps 5 times more potent. Unfortunately, this resulted in the death of various E. Coli germs that are useful in the intestines, vagina, and bladder. The result was an increase in episodes of vaginitis, intestinal upset and resistant organisms.

When the committee met again about 4 years ago, they changed their recommendation. Instead of reverting back to penicillin which is still 99% effective against Strep viridans, they decided to say that there were no evidence-based studies (random, double blind, controlled) upon which to base a judgement. Hence, they sent letters to doctors and dentists saying that SBE prophylaxis is not necessary.

At the bottom of the letter, there was a P.S. stating that people with a birth defect or an artificial valve should probably take something but that the committee could not say what.

The orthopedists are all aware of the danger of Strep viridans getting from the mouth to a prosthetic joint or metal rod. Any foreign body, such as a pacemaker, may be the site where the germs grow.

From my vantage point, for dental work (even cleaning causes bleeding) penicillin pills appear to be safe and effective in combatting Strep viridans.

If one has an operation involving the G1 or GU systems or another system, then consideration should be given to a different antibiotic.

Most people who have heart murmurs have a difference in a valve which would increase their risk of SBE. Therefore, as for over 50 years, penicillin pills before dental work would seem prudent. If one is allergic to penicillin, then erythromycin may be substituted.

Chapter 73: Vertigo Visit

Perhaps thirty years ago, about 2 AM, I was sound asleep when I suddenly awakened with the room spinning out of control like a crazed washing machine. I thought I was going to fall out of bed, so I held on to the mattress until the dizziness reduced a bit and then I crawled to the floor and then the bathroom. About 1 foot from the toilet, I experienced sudden nausea and projectile vomiting. I held my head rigidly still for a number of minutes and then stood up and turned on the light. I could see there was no blood in the vomitus. I decided that meningitis might be a possibility. Hence, I dressed, and quietly went to the hospital. As I walked at a snail's pace through the ER door, I was greeted by one of the physicians, Dr. John Mueller. I told John what had occurred. He took me to an examining room, checked my temperature, BP, my neck, my eyes, and other neurologic signs. Everything seemed normal and I was feeling better with just a bit of dizziness remaining. He was ready to send me home, but I urged him to check a CBC for signs of infection. In a short time (there was no other patient in the ER!), the results came back normal. I was given a prescription for meclizine 25 mg and returned home. I got back into bed and immediately fell asleep. When the alarm clock (a wind-up mechanized clock) went off at 7 AM, I slowly turned to shut it off. There was no dizziness. I was back to normal. It had just been vertigo, not a tumor or meningitis.

Since then I have had 1 episode of vertigo every 10 years. They have been brief and mild. However, I still take my bottle of meclizine with me on vacation, just in case.

Chapter 74: Love at First Hug

Many years ago, I walked into the examining room at the end of the hall to see a new patient. She was an elderly, thin lady, already seated on the examining table. I introduced myself and walked over and shook her hand. She tried to say her name but her speech was severely garbled. She reached out and gave me a big hug. I knew she was my kind of gal. It was love at first hug.

Her daughter was seated in a chair. She quickly told me her mom's name and that she had incurred a stroke recently, while living in another state. She had just moved here to be near her daughter.

Except for her speech, she had recovered well from her stroke. The task at hand was to keep her from having a second one, possibly a fatal one. Her blood pressure was somewhat elevated (140/90) on a low dose vasodilator. She was prescribed a higher dose. She was not on a cholesterol lowering medicine but was begun on Mevacor a few days later after the results of blood tests. She was already on aspirin 325 mg qd.

This lovely lady was always a joy to see. She was smiling every visit and laughed when her daughter teased that I'd better be careful because she might kidnap me. She lived over 10 years more and eventually died of a non-cardiac condition.

The daughter eventually became my patient. She was pleased with the care that her mom received and said she herself wanted to avoid a stroke if at all possible.

Salt reduction, sugar reduction, weight reduction, regular exercise(cardio) 6 times per week, increased fish intake 6 times or more per week, and blood donations to lower iron have been instituted. Screening tests for arteriosclerosis (hardening of the arteries) have been performed. She will be sticking to the program, so her chance of a stroke or heart attack will be greatly reduced.

The daughter has been advised to educate her siblings and get them to undergo screening tests and start a program of risk reduction. A positive family history of stroke or heart attack should be a warning. It used to be considered very important but recent data challenges the importance of family history in someone over the age of 65.

Chapter 75: Lasix

How long does Lasix last? It is a simple question but one in which the most frequent response is: "I don't know."

Lasix is the brand name for generic furosemide, the most common diuretic (water pill) prescribed for congestive heart failure(CHF).

It is called Lasix because it lasts 6 hours, just as it sounds.

Nonetheless, it is most often prescribed in the morning, perhaps 8 AM, in spite of the fact that this is the time of day when most people are at their lowest level of fluid in the body. Most people have not been drinking for eight hours while they are asleep. Most people with unnecessary fluid in the body have been making urine (which they excrete upon waking) while they sleep because their legs are on a level with the kidneys, which has not been the case for most of the day.

The average person with CHF develops increasing edema throughout the day until he or she finally goes to bed and elevates the legs. During the day, most people are sitting or standing and so the fluid is pulled by gravity down to the lower part of the body. The kidneys have no idea that fluid is building up in the legs. But overnight, when the legs are on a level with the kidneys for hours, the fluid migrates up to the kidneys and they are suddenly presented with extra fluid. They decide whether or not the fluid is necessary and recycle it into the bloodstream if it is needed. If the fluid is not needed, it is sent to the bladder to be excreted in the urine. This is called nocturia.

Fifty years ago, the treatment of edema from CHF or kidney failure or eclampsia (kidney failure during pregnancy) was hospitalization with bed rest, elevation of the legs, and fluid and salt restriction. It worked the overwhelming majority of the time.

Nowadays, the hospital beds and the reclining chairs may elevate the knees but not the feet to the level of the kidneys. One almost has to lie down on a bed or couch or on the floor and place pillows under the legs. How much time one spends with the legs elevated depends on how much edema is present.

To have the most benefit, Lasix should be given 6 hours before bedtime in order to rid oneself of extra fluid before bedtime. If one goes to bed at 10 PM, then Lasix would be most helpful around 4 PM. Each person is different. For some, 3 PM might be preferable.

Fifty years ago, many hospital ER admissions would occur at around 11 PM after having dinner at a Chinese restaurant. The proprietors and cooks had determined that people would think the food tasted better with salt and would be thirstier and order more beverages. Previously, a German tavern owner figured out that free salted pretzels at his tavern increased the number of drinks ordered.

There is a misconception that everyone needs 8 glasses of fluid per day. The National Science Foundation declared in

2015 that this was not the case. They discussed the sleep disruption and a staggering number of plastic bottles which require burial and releasing plastic into the environment.

If one urinates 300 cc (10 oz.) and then drinks 500 cc then one overcomes the benefit of diuretics. One needs to have some limitation in the early phase of CHF. One needs to consider ice cream, sherbet, soup, gravy, yogurt, and jello as 99% fluid. We ourselves and most solid foods are about 95% water. One possible fluid limitation is 1200 cc (40 oz.) at the start of treatment with liberalization of intake as treatment progresses.

Tomato juice is to be avoided. Some brands have about 500 mg of sodium in a 4 oz. can. It is amazing that it doesn't drop to the bottom of the container.

CHF is the most frequent DRG diagnosis for first admissions and for repeat admissions in the Medicare age group. The government believes that readmissions are preventable, just like a urinary tract infection, and should warrant a reduction in remuneration.

CHF is extremely complicated and is increasing in prevalence. One factor is the increasing number of people in the Medicare age group. Another is the epidemic of obesity. Some estimates are that 33% of U.S. adult citizens are obese and perhaps 20% in addition are overweight. It is estimated that one pound of fat tissue requires one mile of blood vessels. This is a huge increase in the workload of the heart. Thus, weight reduction of about one pound per week resulting in a fifty-pound weight loss over a year would be of great help in reducing CHF.

CHF is extremely complicated and requires a full-court press with everyone doing his or her part. The following practices may help someone with CHF:

1. Fluid restriction (1200 cc or less)
2. Elevation of legs above kidneys when able (while reading, talking on the phone, watching TV, napping)
3. Salt reduction
4. Weight reduction (1 pound/week)
5. Lasix (furosemide) (lasts 6 hours) should be administered perhaps at 4 PM, additionally at 10 AM if single dose not effective enough
6. Other diuretics if necessary, including spironolactone (holds on to potassium) if potassium is too low and kidney function is normal
7. Lowering of blood pressure if indicated
8. Planning of administration of medicines (if patient is debilitated especially) with pill boxes and daily phone calls from relatives, friends, or health care provider
9. Daily weights in AM before eating after urinating, calling doctor if any two-pound weight gain on same scale since arrival back home
10. May need to weigh at 3 PM if edema reappears; consider calling MD or nurse for guidance related to dosage of lasix

Chapter 76: A Well-Balanced Frame of Mind

While at Shiprock Hospital on the Navajo Reservation from 1973 to 1975, there were a number of patients who likely had terminal cancer and some who were depressed. In arranging a course on Navajo culture for other Anglo (as we were called on a good day) healthcare providers, I had met and inquired of a medicine man, called a singer, as to the appropriateness of having a sing, or cleansing ceremony, in the hospital. I was told that it would be somewhat limited but ok, with the understanding that a full ceremony be performed later outside the hospital. Consequently, I suggested to a few patients that they have a sing in the hospital. I did not attend but I could later see that it was beneficial for the patient and the family.

There are a number of different sings which range in duration from one to seven days and are supervised in detail by a singer who has spent years learning approximately three ceremonies. The singer must memorize words, songs, motions, use paraphernalia and plants, and create a sand painting on the ground. It's more complicated than an opera.

The goal of a sing is to restore balance to a person's life when something is amiss – an imbalance with one's family, friends, community, the earth, the sky, the flora, or fauna, in effect the universe. Native American spirituality is called animism.

One may learn more from a book entitled Code Talker by Chester Nez. He grew up south of Gallup, New Mexico, and was educated at schools that forbade the speaking of Navajo. As a teenager, he volunteered for the marines during World War II and was one of approximately thirty Navajo who were ordered to create a code using Navajo words. The Japanese were never able to break this code. It saved thousands of lives in the Pacific theatre including Guadalcanal and Iwo Jima. Chester Nez and his cohort of 400 Navajo Code Talkers were forbidden to disclose the existence of the code, even with their families, until 1966. How ironic that a Native American tribe that was targeted for extinction and with the intent of destroying their language should use their forbidden words to save so many lives and play such a critical part in protecting our country.

Chapter 77: Things Can Get Squirrelly When Something Seems Trivial

There was a lady who came from Pennsylvania to have her coronary arteries ballooned(PTCA). She was having persistent chest pain, angina, which was relieved following the PTCA.

Two years later, she drove all the way here to the ER with chest pain that was continuous but with some waxing and waning of discomfort. Her vital signs were normal as were her EKG's and blood tests. NTG sublingually did not help; nor did pain pills.

I did not know what the cause of pain was so I consulted a pain management physician to see if he could help. He inquired about exposure to deer. The patient said that she did not come near deer but she had this cute little squirrel that she had tamed. My colleague ordered Lyme titres which were abnormal. He started antibiotics and the pain resolved.

Years ago, in Ann Arbor, as a resident in medicine, I had admitted an 80-year-old man through the ER with a high fever, kidney failure, and liver failure. Part of my evaluation included questions such as: "Have you done anything unusual lately?" "Have you made contact with any pets including parakeets?" The gentleman had recently cleaned out a squirrel's nest in his garage. His temperature actually increased with IV penicillin. Two weeks later, complicated blood titres confirmed what I had suspected. He had an illness called leptospirosis which was present in squirrel excrement and was cured with penicillin.

There is no question that is too trivial.

Chapter 78: The Dog Ate My Scale

A sixty-year old gentleman came for a visit for high blood pressure, high cholesterol, and obesity. He was a teacher who had dutifully kept his appointments over a number of years.

After inquiring about his symptoms, he was examined and then weighed. His weight was a bit higher this visit just as it had been in the past: an undesirable upward trend.

I again reviewed his particular risks including high blood pressure, elevated triglycerides, overweight, low HDL and elevated blood sugar (pre-diabetes) which placed him in a category called Metabolic Syndrome. It is a pre-diabetic condition that increases the risk of heart attack, stroke, and dementia by 30%.

Previously it was recommended that he try to focus on these issues and lose a half a pound to a pound per week by reducing his calorie intake by 100 calories per day. He could give up a glass of orange juice, milk, soft drink, or alcohol. It would not even warrant the use of the heinous label, DIET. A majority of people can lose weight simply by reducing the number of calorie-containing beverages they drink. Water, tea and Crystal Lite are good substitutes.

As a first step toward improving focus and changing suboptimal eating (and drinking) habits, it is usually recommended that a patient keep a record of his or her weight on a daily basis and show me the list on the next visit. I asked this patient if he had kept a WEIGHT list. I expected a response such as, "I left the list in the car," or "We just moved 6 months ago and we can't find the scale."

Instead, the patient treated me to the following explanation: "Doc, you're not going to believe this but my dog ate my scale." I could not help but laugh and remarked that I wish I had a nickel for each time one of his students must have used the time-honored old excuse that the "dog ate my homework." Didn't he feel just a bit silly?

I asked if he owned a Great Dane or a St. Bernard or a Rotweiler. His response: "a chihuahua mutt." I asked when this tragic event occurred and had the dog recovered from eating 5 pounds of plastic and metal. The patient started to choke a little in his response to me but was able to state: "Six months ago, and it's still going on." I strongly suggested that he throw the scale or the dog out before the dog died and an autopsy revealed high levels of aluminum. The ASPCA would not let this slip past them. I could just see the newspaper headline, "Teacher Kills Pet Dog with Scaled-Down Diet!"

Chapter 79: A-Pop-Toe-Sis

No, this is not a test for Alzheimers to see if you can remember these words 5 minutes later (but it could be). The word, APOPTOSIS, means cell death at an unexpected rate or time. It is easier to remember A-Pop-Toe-Sis if one thinks about his sister trying a ballet pirouette when her big toe on the right foot pops out of joint. Ouch!

Over the years many patients have told me that they have enjoyed perfect health until some untoward event occurs, and then all of a sudden they learn that 3, 4, or 5 organs are in bad shape. They would like an explanation to this puzzling conundrum of why they are all-of-a-sudden falling apart.

Many, many years ago, a thoughtful physician named Oliver Wendell Holmes Sr. offered an explanation in his wonderful poem entitled, “The Deacon’s Carriage,” or, “The Wonderful One-Hoss Shay.” He describes how this carriage-maker figured out what were the best materials, including various kinds of wood, leather, and metal, to use to create the best, most long-lasting carriage.

The carriage was user-friendly and without breakage of any kind for 100 years. Then one day various parts of the carriage started to split and break. The metal parts were rusting. The leather parts were rotting. Within a short period of time the carriage was done. Repairs would only prolong the inevitable: the scrap yard. The carriage-maker had created a marvel of function and appearance, but it was fated to last just a certain number of years.

Presently, we are extending the life expectancy with a multitude of weapons at our disposal: medications, procedures, operations, artificial parts, pacemakers, defibrillators, transplants, targeted therapies for cancer, and immune diseases, stem cells, gene therapies, etc...

There are studies underway now to clarify what determines the rate of apoptosis. At some point we will be able to slow the rate of aging itself. Regardless, death seems to be inevitable. As individuals, we need to maintain healthy habits (regular exercise, weight control, avoiding salt, man-made sugars, and fats, eating more fish, utilizing screening tests, taking prescribed medicines as prescribed) and live each day with the knowledge that it may be our last. Health should be a priority. It is not a given. We are not entitled to good health or a long life. We must choose what is best for us and not be dictated to by our taste buds.

There is ample evidence that our species is the smartest on the planet. There is also strong evidence that we are the least intelligent. What other species fails from day one to teach its progeny about what is safe and also what are the best foods? We have substituted a lot of our instinctive "intelligence" with a modicum of free will. Sometimes we need a good kick in the pants from our parents or elders. In this technological age, this would probably be labelled, "rebooting."

The quality and length of life can be improved upon with good decision-making. Keep your shay strong!.

Chapter 80: Ethics: A Slippery Slope; A State of Mind

Recently I attended a session of the Virginia Bar Association on ethical issues surrounding death. It was well attended and wide ranging in questions posed.

It reminded me of a session in 1970 in medical school that Joseph Fletcher, the UVA ethicist, conducted in our small apartment on Oakhurst Circle. Fletcher labelled his approach to ethical issues as Situation Ethics. In essence as I remember it, his approach was to treat each situation as unique and view things with an open mind regardless of the particular organizational credos of the patient or our own religious beliefs. Tolerance and maintaining the health of the patient as the number one priority were emphasized.

One of my medical school classmates is an ace of person who exudes the milk of human kindness. Early on she took a group of us students to the movies to see Gone With the Wind. She brought a box of Kleenex which she freely shared. She started to cry during the overture. I think she believed that the South should have won the Civil War. She told us that she herself had never left the state of Virginia.

Later on, at an ethics session, we were asked about our attitude toward treating someone's health problem, perhaps venereal disease, if they had different beliefs. Our truly wonderful classmate volunteered that her religion taught that homosexuality was a sin. She would feel that she should treat the person but also be compelled to tell him that he was committing a sin.

Another classmate offered the opinion that this would be imposing one's beliefs on the patient and might not be best. Years later our ace of hearts went across state lines, met and married a gentleman from Morocco who is Jewish, converted to Judaism, and keeps kosher at home in Miami. Love rules! Where love rules, tolerance flourishes.

Chapter 81: Pillars of Medicine

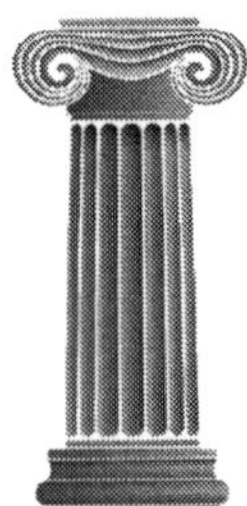

1. Do no harm:
   a. Avoid errors of commission: question risks of treatment or recommendations formed for a population of patients as opposed to individualizing treatment.
   b. Avoid errors of omission: beware of backing off from appropriate treatment due to fear of criticism.

2. Continuity of Care: get to know your patient, establish a rapport, discuss goals, create a happy relationship, build trust. Get to know your patient's mannerisms. Be on the alert for subtle changes in status.

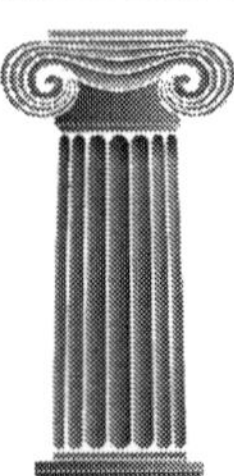

3. Treat each person as a unique individual. Recommend same treatment as for your mother.

Not necessarily a panel algorithm

Listen to the patient

Explain problems, choices, recommendations, in lay terms

Be honest, straight forward

Be available

Be consistent

Be compassionate, caring, empathetic and loving

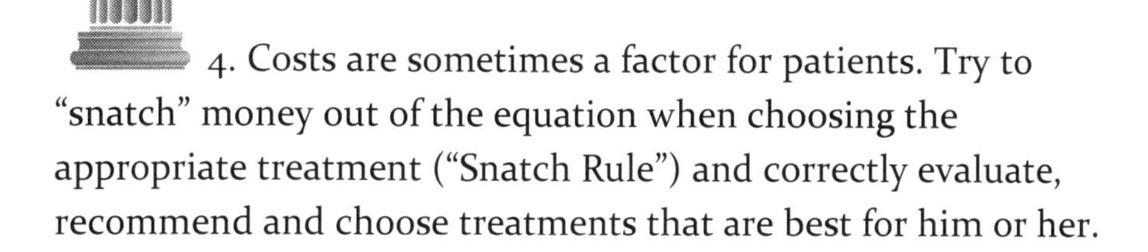

4. Costs are sometimes a factor for patients. Try to "snatch" money out of the equation when choosing the appropriate treatment ("Snatch Rule") and correctly evaluate, recommend and choose treatments that are best for him or her.

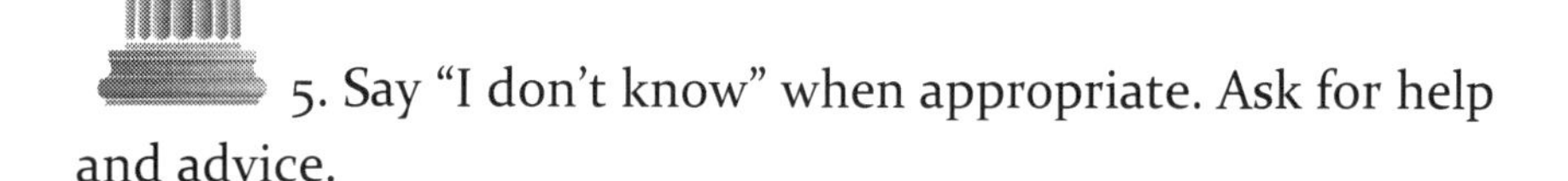

5. Say "I don't know" when appropriate. Ask for help and advice.

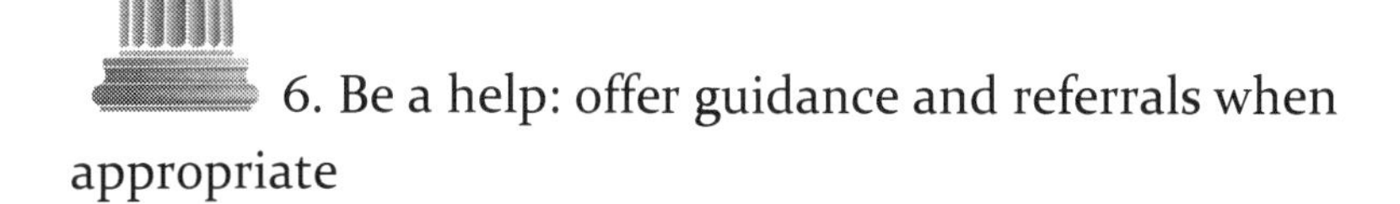

6. Be a help: offer guidance and referrals when appropriate

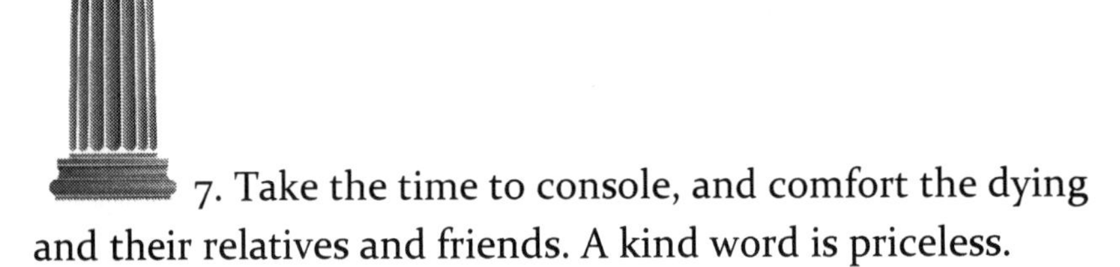

7. Take the time to console, and comfort the dying and their relatives and friends. A kind word is priceless.

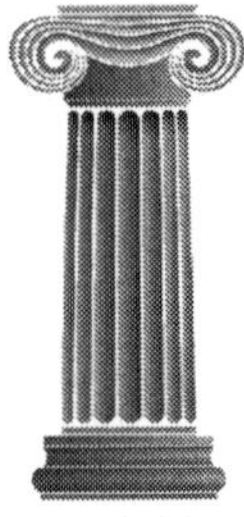

8. Provide care to those in need whether low or no income, or no insurance.

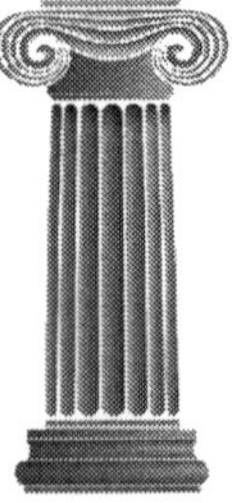

9. Keep an open mind: question accepted beliefs. Think.

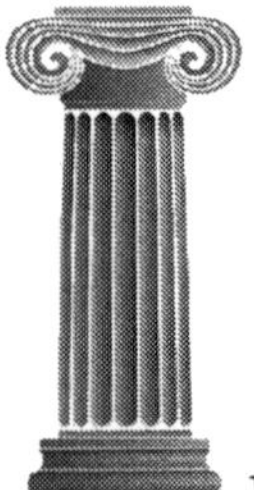

10. Take responsibility for your patient. Try to provide appropriate care.

Chapter 82: Change is Constant

Everything changes. Nothing stays the same. Healthcare itself is changing rapidly with many new medications, robotic surgery, immunotherapies, and use of genetic information, to name but a few discoveries and innovations. I, myself, have been the beneficiary of new therapies.

The practice of medicine is changing rapidly. Fewer than 1% of graduating medical students are choosing primary care, pediatrics, family practice, or general internal medicine.

Our country only graduates approximately 13,000 medical students per year. We take in about 13,000 foreign medical graduates per year. There is no pre-selection for tuition or stipends in exchange for a promise to serve in a needy area for an extended period, except perhaps through the military or isolated programs. In spite of an increasingly older population of patients, Medicare Part B is budgeting less and less, so that physician reimbursement is around 12% of the healthcare pie. Government leaders and policy analysts are calling lowered physician reimbursement "value based care" as though cost cutting is possible because previously, care given was often not necessary, inappropriate and money driven. (If the theory is that fee for service meant physicians would provide care based on how much more money they'd receive instead of what they believed would help the patient, isn't the assumption ironic or contradictory that value-based care, lowering reimbursement, means the care physicians do *not* provide in the future is only based on correct medical appraisal and not because it would be unpaid care? Pause and ponder that. I think reimbursement theories and assumptions should not be swallowed whole but tested if we truly want patients to get the right care.)

Another inconsistency is that hospitals, according to a government report, are paid up to significantly more than doctors in private practice for the very same services. Hence, hospitals are able to employ doctors, bill and collect for the services at a significantly higher rate, pay doctors a salary, and keep the difference or reduce their salaries when contracts come due (unless prohibited by contract.)

Pharmaceutical companies are given patents for years and then may get new patents if the medicine is altered slightly. Their lobby might dissuade our government from limiting how the companies charge for medicines, unlike the case for physician and hospital services. (However, the Canadian government refuses to pay more than 30 cents on the dollar for US-made medicines and the companies accept this.)

We are moving more quickly toward a socialist system with a single payer. Almost all doctors will be employees, not employers. Most hospitals are already run by administrators, not doctors. Tensions can and do arise at times between medical staff and administration about patient care. Building a teamwork mentality requires mutual respect and shared values. Hospitals do have to survive. For the doctors, their legal and ethical duty should always be to the patient based on the best medical information available to them.

Doctors are presently in large numbers working in shifts. There is little discussion of the pillars of medicine: continuity of care, a close doctor patient relationship, or recommending the same treatment you would recommend for your mother. If you would like to know more about the realities of a socialized medical system, I would recommend Henry Marsh's book Do No Harm (noted earlier). Dr. Marsh describes how his admissions and operations are delayed and cancelled because of necessary personnel going home at a set time and rules that a bed be empty in the ICU before an operation is begun. But Dr. Marsh also beautifully describes the joy of being a doctor and taking care of patients, in spite of a dysfunctional system.

I, myself, am ecstatic about having become a doctor, helping people whenever I can, and continuing to learn and to grow. I would make the same choices regarding going to medical school, experiencing internship, residency, and fellowship. I would recommend a career in medicine to anyone who enjoys people, wants to keep learning and work hard, to be challenged and make a difference every day. I hope the next generation of healthcare providers will realize what a privilege and a joy being a physician can be. It is a calling and not a job. I hope this book will cause the reader to smile a bit and encourage physicians to be faithful guardians of their patients' hopes and health.

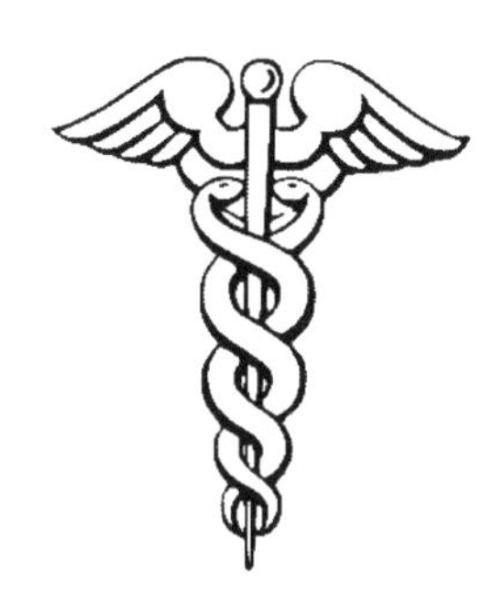

And now, as in real life, reluctantly, I must accede to my wife having the last word.

Post Script

Upon reading the last chapter and paragraph of Bill's opus, as he calls it, I recalled a recent moment. Two years ago, I attended some meetings in Charlottesville, Virginia; we were headquartered in a hotel right across from the old medical school entrance. Very early one morning, I stepped out alone onto the hotel patio that overlooked a narrow side street below. The street led up to the old medical school Bill had attended. In the hush and dim light of early morning, I spotted a lone figure moving down the street toward the school. It was a young male, carrying books or laptop under one arm and wearing the telltale short white jacket that third and fourth year medical students wore back in Bill's day. The student moved quickly and with purpose, not lagging with fatigue or lack of energy. A sense of something like excitement was almost palpable. I looked closer and for a moment my heart leapt as I imagined it was Bill as I remembered him from so many years ago, energetically heading off to his studies to become a doctor. Quickly recovering the reality of the moment, I wiped away a surprising tear. Then I wished that whoever the young student below was, he would find the same joy, luck, and satisfaction as Bill has found taking care of patients.

We need that.

Made in the USA
Middletown, DE
10 February 2018